Statistics for Biology and Health

Series Editors:
M. Gail
K. Krickeberg
J. Samet
A. Tsiatis
W. Wong

For other titles published in this series, go to
http://www.springer.com/series/2848

Toshiro Tango

Statistical Methods for Disease
Clustering

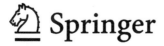 Springer

Toshiro Tango
Department of Technology Assesment & Biostatistics
National Institute of Public Health
3-6 Minami 2 chome
Wako, Saitama
351-0197 Japan
tango@niph.go.jp

Editors:

M. Gail
National Cancer Institute
Bethesda, MD 20892
USA

K. Krickeberg
Le Chatelet
F-63270 Manglieu
France

Jonathan M. Samet
Department of Preventive Medicine
Keck School of Medicine
University of Southern California
1441 Eastlake Ave. Room 4436, MC 9175
Los Angeles, CA 90089
USA

A. Tsiatis
Department of Statistics
North Carolina State University
Raleigh, NC 27695
USA

W. Wong
Department of Statistics
Stanford University
Stanford, CA 94305-4065
USA

ISSN 1431-8776
ISBN 978-1-4419-1571-9   e-ISBN 978-1-4419-1572-6
DOI 10.1007/978-1-4419-1572-6
Springer New York Dordrecht Heidelberg London

Library of Congress Control Number: 2010920016

© Springer Science+Business Media, LLC 2010
All rights reserved. This work may not be translated or copied in whole or in part without the written permission of the publisher (Springer Science+Business Media, LLC, 233 Spring Street, New York, NY 10013, USA), except for brief excerpts in connection with reviews or scholarly analysis. Use in connection with any form of information storage and retrieval, electronic adaptation, computer software, or by similar or dissimilar methodology now known or hereafter developed is forbidden.
The use in this publication of trade names, trademarks, service marks, and similar terms, even if they are not identified as such, is not to be taken as an expression of opinion as to whether or not they are subject to proprietary rights.

Printed on acid-free paper

Springer is part of Springer Science+Business Media (www.springer.com)

Preface

This book is intended to provide a text on statistical methods for detecting clusters and/or clustering of health events that is of interest to final-year undergraduate- and graduate-level statistics, biostatistics, epidemiology, and geography students but will also be of relevance to public health practitioners, statisticians, biostatisticians, epidemiologists, medical geographers, human geographers, environmental scientists, and ecologists. Prerequisites are introductory biostatistics and epidemiology courses.

With increasing public health concerns about environmental risks, the need for sophisticated methods for analyzing spatial health events is immediate. Furthermore, the research area of statistical tests for disease clustering now attracts a wide audience due to the perceived need to implement wide-ranging monitoring systems to detect possible health-related bioterrorism activity. With this background and the development of the geographical information system (GIS), the analysis of disease clustering of health events has seen considerable development over the last decade. Therefore, several excellent books on spatial epidemiology and statistics have recently been published. However, it seems to me that there is no other book solely focusing on statistical methods for disease clustering. I hope that readers will find this book useful and interesting as an introduction to the subject.

Although the view of statistical methods of disease clustering embodied in this book is, of course, my own, it has been formed over many years through collaboration and contact with many statisticians. Especially, I must acknowledge the tremendous debt I owe to Martin Kulldorff, who has always provided me with invaluable insight and suggestions for improving my original ideas. I also thank Kunihiko Takahashi for preparing several figures and carefully reading the final text. My thanks also go to John Kimmel of Springer for inviting me to write this book and providing continual support and encouragement. Finally, I would like to thank Taeko Becque for checking my poor English.

Tokyo

Toshiro Tango
July 2009

Contents

1 Introduction 1
  1.1 Classification of Disease Clustering 2
  1.2 Data Used for Disease Clustering 4
  1.3 Organization of the Book 5
  1.4 Organization of the Chapters 5
  1.5 Statistical Software 6
    1.5.1 R 6
    1.5.2 SaTScan 6
    1.5.3 FleXScan 7
    1.5.4 Splancs 7

2 Clustering and Clusters 9
  2.1 Spatial Pattern 9
  2.2 Spatial Point Process...................................... 12
    2.2.1 Homogeneous Poisson Process 12
    2.2.2 Inhomogeneous Poisson Process 14
  2.3 Back to the Questions 14
  2.4 Approaches Using Regional Count Data 15
  2.5 Approaches Using Case-Control Location Data 25
  2.6 Monte Carlo Hypothesis Testing 29
  2.7 Spatial Autocorrelation 30

3 Disease Mapping: Visualization of
Spatial Clustering 33
  3.1 Standardization 35
  3.2 Basic Models for Relative Risk 38
  3.3 Likelihood Models 39
  3.4 Poisson-Gamma Bayesian Models 40
    3.4.1 Empirical Bayes Estimator 41
    3.4.2 Hierarchical Full Bayes Estimator 42
  3.5 Hierarchical Bayesian Models 44

     3.5.1   Log-normal Model 44
     3.5.2   Conditional Autoregressive Model 46

4   Tests for Temporal Clustering 49
   4.1   Data.. 51
   4.2   Null Hypothesis vs. Alternative Hypothesis 51
   4.3   Historical Overview of Methods 52
   4.4   Selected Methods 55
     4.4.1   Ederer-Myers-Mantel's Method for Count Data 56
     4.4.2   Naus' Scan Statistic for Point Data 57
     4.4.3   Nagarwalla's Scan Statistic for Point Data 58
     4.4.4   Kulldorff's Scan Statistic for Count Data 59
     4.4.5   Tango's Index for Count Data 60
   4.5   Illustration with Real Data 62
     4.5.1   Congenital Oesophageal Atresia Data 62
     4.5.2   Trisomy Data 68
   4.6   Discussion 69

5   General Tests for Spatial Clustering: Regional Count Data......... 71
   5.1   Data.. 73
   5.2   Null Hypothesis vs. Alternative Hypothesis 73
   5.3   Historical Overview of Methods 75
   5.4   Selected Methods 86
     5.4.1   Tango's Index for Spatial Clustering 86
     5.4.2   Kulldorff's Circular Spatial Scan Statistic 88
     5.4.3   Tango and Takahashi's Flexible Spatial Scan Statistic 89
     5.4.4   Tango's Spatial Scan Statistic with Restricted Likelihood
           Ratio 90
   5.5   Illustration with Real Data 91
     5.5.1   Japanese Gallbladder Cancer Mortality Data 91
     5.5.2   New York Incident Leukemia Cases..................... 100
   5.6   Power Comparison 102

6   General Tests for Spatial Clustering : Case-Control Point Data 113
   6.1   Data.. 115
   6.2   Null Hypothesis vs. Alternative Hypothesis 115
   6.3   Historical Overview of Methods 116
   6.4   Selected Methods 119
     6.4.1   Cuzick and Edwards' Test 119
     6.4.2   Tango's Index for Spatial Clustering 121
     6.4.3   Diggle and Chetwynd's Test 125
     6.4.4   Kulldorff's Spatial Scan Statistic 128
   6.5   Illustration with Real Data 129
     6.5.1   Leukemia and lymphoma in North Humberside 129
     6.5.2   Early Medieval Grave Sites 139

6.6   Discussion 146

7   Tests for Space-Time Clustering 149
  7.1   Data... 150
  7.2   Null Hypothesis vs Alternative Hypothesis 150
  7.3   Historical Overview of Methods 151
  7.4   Selected Methods 160
      7.4.1   Knox's Test 160
      7.4.2   Mantel's Test....................................... 161
      7.4.3   Baker's Max Test for the Knox Test 162
      7.4.4   Jacquez's *k*-NN Test................................ 163
      7.4.5   Diggle *et al.*'s Test 164
      7.4.6   Kulldorff and Hjalmars's Approach for the Knox Test...... 167
  7.5   Illustrations with Real Data 168
      7.5.1   Kaposi's Sarcoma in the West Nile Distric of Uganda 168
  7.6   Power Comparison 178

8   Focused Tests for Spatial Clustering 181
  8.1   Data... 182
  8.2   Null Hypothesis vs. Alternative Hypothesis.................... 183
  8.3   Historical Overview of Methods 185
  8.4   Selected Methods 191
      8.4.1   Stone's Test 191
      8.4.2   Bithell's Linear Risk Score Test 192
      8.4.3   Waller and Lawson's Score Test 192
      8.4.4   Tango's Score Test for Decline Trend 193
      8.4.5   Tango's Score Test for Peak-Decline Trend.............. 194
      8.4.6   Diggle, Morris, and Morton-Jones' Test Based on
              Case-Control Point Data 195
  8.5   Illustration with Real Data 196
      8.5.1   Infant Deaths Around Municipal Solid Waste Incinerators .. 196
      8.5.2   Leukemia Cases Near Inactive Hazardous Waste Sites 203
      8.5.3   Larynx and Lung Cancer Near a Disused Incinerator....... 204
  8.6   Power Comparison 205

9   Space-Time Scan Statistics 211
  9.1   Data... 211
  9.2   Null Hypothesis vs. Alternative Hypothesis.................... 213
  9.3   Historical Overview of Methods 214
      9.3.1   Retrospective Analysis.............................. 215
      9.3.2   Syndromic Surveillance............................. 216
  9.4   Selected Methods 219
      9.4.1   Kulldorff's Cylindrical Space-Time Scan Statistic 219
      9.4.2   Takahashi *et al.*'s Prismatic Space-time Scan Statistic 220
  9.5   Illustration with Real Data 221

9.5.1   Syndromic Surveillance of the Massachusetts Data 222
9.6   Power Comparison 224
9.7   Discussion with a New Proposal 224

A   List of R functions 235
     References 236

Index 245

Chapter 1

Introduction

In epidemiological studies, it is often of importance to evaluate whether a disease is randomly distributed or tends to occur as clusters over time and/or space after adjusting for known confounding factors, that may provide clues to the etiology of the disease. There has recently been great public concern about clustering of health events such as the occurrence of childhood leukemia, birth defects, and cancer. For example, since the early 1960s, it has been argued that childhood leukemia could be caused by either an infectious agent or an environmental toxin. Therefore, many researchers have examined space-time clustering of childhood leukemias in relation to the date and place of onset or diagnosis using various methods, including the Knox test. Furthermore, since the 1980s, there has been growing interest in the relation between the risk of a disease and proximity of residence to a prespecified putative source of hazard. It is well-known that the apparent excess of cases of childhood leukemia near a nuclear reprocessing plant such as that in the village near Seascale facility at Sellafield has been extensively investigated (for example, see Bithell *et al.*, 1994). More recently, there has been great public concern about the health effects of *dioxins*, organic compounds such as polychlorinated dibenzodioxins (PCDDs) and dibenzofurans (PCDFs), emitted from municipal solid waste incinerators (for example, see Elliott *et al.*, 1996).

In 1990, the Centers for Disease Control and Prevention (1990a, 1990b) issued the "Guidelines for investigating clusters of health events". In its appendix (1990b), a "summary of methods for statistically assessing clusters of health events" is provided as a resource for investigators who may become involved with the statistical aspect of *reported clusters* of health events.

In this book, I would like to introduce statistical methods for detecting disease clustering and/or localized clusters that are widely used and/or widely known in the literature and illustrate them with several real data sets. Almost all of the methods introduced here are used for *retrospective analysis*, except for the methods for syndromic surveillance in Chapter 9.

T. Tango, *Statistical Methods for Disease Clustering*,
Statistics for Biology and Health, DOI 10.1007/978-1-4419-1572-6_1,
© Springer Science+Business Media, LLC 2010

1.1 Classification of Disease Clustering

Disease clustering is classified into one of three groups: *temporal clustering*, *spatial clustering*, or *space-time clustering*.

- *Temporal clustering* examines the question of whether cases tend to be located close to each other in time. One article illustrates this:

> An outbreak of acute nonbacterial gastroenteritis occurred among residents and staff in a nursing home in Baltimore, Maryland, in December 1980. A total of 101 residents and 69 staff members were surveyed by question-naire. The attack rate (defined as acute onset of vomiting or two or more loose stools per 24 hours) was 46% of the group. Illness was brief and mild; no patients were hospitalized, and there were no deaths. Person-to-person transmission was documented by **temporal clustering** of cases (the demonstration of a higher rate of illness among residents exposed to an ill roommate one or two days earlier than among those not similarly exposed. ... The analysis of **temporal clustering** of cases was particularly useful in documenting person-to-person transmission in this outbreak and might be used for this purpose in other outbreaks caused by Norwalk or Norwalk-like viruses, as well as in outbreaks associated with other infectious organisms (Kaplan *et al.*, *American Journal of Epidemiology* 1982; **116**:940–948).

- *Spatial clustering* examines the question of whether cases tend to be located close to each other in space.
- *Space-time clustering* examines the question of whether cases that are close in space are also close in time. The following study illustrates this:

> The authors analyzed the natural history of multiple sclerosis (MS) be-fore onset to identify the period of susceptibility and exogenous factors that might play a role in causing the disease. **Space-time cluster analy-sis** was performed among northern Sardinians, a genetically stable Italian population that showed an increasing risk of MS between 1965 and 1999. Residence changes from birth to clinical onset were recorded for all MS patients with clinical onset between 1965 and 1999 in the province of Sas-sari. ... **Clustering** was substantial in early childhood. **Clustering** was most marked in the most recent cases, among women, and among patients with early age at onset, a relapsing-remitting course, and in the eastern subarea... (Pugliatti *et al.*, *American Journal of Epidemiology* 2006; **164**:326–333).

To investigate whether clustering is real and significant, many different tests have been proposed for different purposes. Besag and Newell (1991) classified these tests into two families:

- *General tests* designed for investigating the question of whether clustering occurs over the study region.
- *Focused tests* designed for assessing the clustering around a pre-fixed point such as a nuclear installation. The following study illustrates this:

> Some recent epidemiologic studies suggest an association between lymphatic and hematopoietic cancers and residential exposure to high-frequency electromagnetic fields (100 kHz to 300 GHz) generated by radio and television transmitters. Vatican Radio is a very powerful station located in a northern suburb of Rome, Italy. In the 10-km area around the station, with 49,656 residents (in 1991), leukemia mortality among adults (aged > 14 years; 40 cases) in 1987–1998 and childhood leukemia incidence (eight cases) in 1987–1999 were evaluated. The risk of childhood leukemia was higher than expected for distances up to 6 km from the radio station (standardized incidence rate = 2.2, 95% confidence interval: 1.0, 4.1), and **there was a significant decline in risk with increasing distance** both for male mortality ($p = 0.03$) and childhood leukemia ($p = 0.036$) (Michelozzi *et al.*, *American Journal of Epidemiology* 2002;**155**:1096–1103).

General tests were further classified by Kulldorff (1998) into two types:

- *Global clustering tests* designed for evaluating whether cases tend to come in groups or are located close to each other no matter when and where they occur. The following study illustrates this:

> A retrospective population-based case-control interview study has been conducted in three distinct areas in the north of England where local excesses of children with leukemia have been reported. A total of 109 cases of childhood (0–14 years at diagnosis) leukemia and non-Hodgkin's lymphoma who were born in one of the study areas and diagnosed there between 1974 and 1988 were included in the study. One control per case was matched on sex, date -of- birth, and health district of birth. **The objective was to compare residential histories of cases and controls and in particular to determine whether case children had lived in the same place at the same time more often than controls.** The residential distance between two children was taken to be the smallest geographical distance between homes they had "occupied" simultaneously for a period of at least six months between conception and diagnosis. **Case children were more likely than expected to have other cases as their nearest neighbors by residential distance** (observed = 69, expected = 54.5, $p = 0.006$) (Alexander *et al.*, *British Journal of Cancer* 1992; **65**:583–588).

- *Cluster detection tests* designed both for detecting localized clusters and evaluating their significance. The following article illustrates this:

> School immunization requirements are important in controlling vaccine-preventable diseases in the United States. Forty-eight states offer nonmedical exemptions to school immunization requirements. Children with exemptions are at increased risk of contracting and transmitting vaccine-preventable diseases. The clustering of nonmedical exemptions can affect a community's risk of vaccine-preventable diseases. The authors evaluated **spatial clustering** of nonmedical exemptions in Michigan and geographic overlap between exemption clusters and clusters of reported pertussis cases. **Kulldorff's scan statistic** identified 23 statistically **significant census tract clusters** for exemption rates and 6 **significant census tract clusters** for reported pertussis cases between 1993 and 2004 (Omer *et al.*, *American Journal of Epidemiology* 2008;**168**:1389–1396).

1.2 Data Used for Disease Clustering

It is probably no exaggeration to say that the cluster investigation started to explore space-time clustering of childhood leukemia in the mid 1960s, when Knox's test (1964a, 1964b) and Mantel's test (1967) were applied. To test for disease clustering, we generally need to collect data retrospectively on the *time of occurrence* and/or the *location* of each case for a defined geographic region during a specified study period. *Date of onset, date of birth*, and *date of death* have been used as the time of occurrence for clustering of childhood leukemia. The rationale for using date of onset invokes a short time interval between the inductive event and onset of disease. A search for clustering by date of birth invokes the hypothesis that childhood leukemias are determined pre- and perinatally, when the human organism is particularly susceptible to the effects of a carcinogen. Needless to say, very great care is required for clustering by date of death because of the long and variable interval between the onset and death. *Address at onset, address at birth*, and *address at death* can be used as the *location* depending on the study objectives. Examples of data used to explore space-time clustering of childhood leukemia are shown below:

Onset cluster: Klauber and Mustacchi (1970) investigated space-time clustering for *time of diagnosis* and address of 149 leukemia cases in children under the age of 15 years diagnosed in San Francisco during the 20-year period 1946 to 1965.
Birth cluster: Klauber (1968) conducted a study of clustering of childhood leukemia by *hospital of birth* where 234 children under age 5 who died of leukemia and who were born during 1958–1960 in California were identified.
Death cluster: Glass and Mantel (1969) analyzed dates and residence data for 298 Los Angeles childhood leukemia deaths during the period 1960–1964.

Data types used for cluster investigation, on the other hand, are generally classified into two types:

- *Individual geographical location data* include data on coordinates of birth, residence, workplace, and death, which are usually residential addresses such as street address, zip code, and post code unit.
- *Regional count data* include the number of cases and population at risk in some small areas usually defined for administrative purposes, such as census tracts, counties, municipalities, and electoral wards.

Due to the restriction of clinical confidentiality, it is often impossible to obtain individual data, and so we have to resort to an analysis of the count within an administrative region.

1.3 Organization of the Book

Chapters 2 and 3 provide readers with a brief introduction to basic concepts of *clustering* and *clusters* and the basic idea of how to detect clustering and disease mapping, which are useful tools for visualizing the *clustering* and *clusters* before going into the details of statistical tests. The remaining chapters are arranged according to the particular type of disease clustering. The book is organized as follows:

- Chapter 2 introduces to the basic concepts of *clustering* and *clusters* and the basic idea of how to detect clustering and/or clusters.
- Chapter 3 introduces to basic concepts of disease mapping and a range of mapping methods that are useful tools for visualizing regional variations of disease risk or regional clustering and/or clusters.
- Chapter 4 presents tests for detecting temporal clustering.
- Chapter 5 discusses general tests for detecting spatial clustering based on regional count data.
- Chapter 6 gives general tests for detecting spatial clustering based on case-control location data.
- Chapter 7 gives tests for space-time clustering or space-time interaction.
- Chapter 8 discusses focused tests for spatial clustering.
- Chapter 9 discusses the space-time scan statistic with special emphasis on the application to a syndromic surveillance.

1.4 Organization of the Chapters

Each of Chapters 4 through 9 has the following basic structure:

- Each chapter begins with illustrative real examples that are later analyzed by some of the selected methods.

- The *Data* section describes the data necessary for cluster investigation and the notation used throughout the chapter.
- The *Null Hypothesis vs. Alternative Hypothesis* section describes the null hypothesis and alternative hypothesis both nonstatistically and statistically.
- The *Historical Overview of Methods* section gives an overview of the *major* methods proposed so far and is not a review of all the methods. So, readers should note that there are several other proposed methods not mentioned here. Furthermore, readers who are not interested in the history can skip this section.
- The *Selected Methods* section describes the details of selected methods, most of which are widely known and/or widely used.
- The *Illustration with Real Data* section illustrates the selected methods with real data sets.
- The *Power Comparison* section compares the powers of the selected methods.
- The *Discussion* section discusses the appropriateness and the relative merits of the methods. This section is generally provided when the *Power Comparison* section could not be set.

1.5 Statistical Software

In each of Chapters 4 through 9, selected methods for detecting disease clustering are illustrated with real data in the *Illustration with Real Data* section using some of the software packages listed below, which are available free of charge. In particular, in the appendix, I provide readers with R functions for some selected methods for ease of applying the methods.

1.5.1 R

URL: http://www.r-project.org/

R is a language and environment for statistical computing and graphics. It is a GNU project that is similar to the S language and environment which was developed at Bell Laboratories (formerly AT&T) by John Chambers and colleagues. R can be considered a different implementation of S. There are some important differences, but much code written for S runs unaltered under R (see the *Introduction to R*).

1.5.2 SaTScan

URL: http://www.satscan.org/

SaTScan is free software that analyzes spatial, temporal, and space-time data using the spatial, temporal, or space-time scan statistics. It is designed for any of the following interrelated purposes:

- To perform geographical surveillance of disease, detect spatial or space-time disease clusters, and see if they are statistically significant.
- To test whether a disease is randomly distributed over space, time, or space and time.
- To evaluate the statistical significance of disease cluster alarms.
- To perform repeated time-periodic disease surveillance for early detection of disease outbreaks.

1.5.3 FleXScan

URL: http://www.niph.go.jp/soshiki/gijutsu/download/flexscan/index_e.html

FlexScan is free software developed to analyze spatial count data using the flexible spatial scan statistic and circular spatial scan statistic. The current version includes a spatial scan statistic with a restricted likelihood ratio. These scan statistics are introduced in Chapter 5. FLeXScan is similar to SaTScan, but the current version of FleXScan is still restricted to spatial analyses.

1.5.4 Splancs

URL: http://www.maths.lancs.ac.uk/rowlings/Splancs/

Splancs is a software package for spatial and space-time point pattern analysis (Rowlingson and Diggle, 1993) that can be installed in R. See also Bivand and Gebhardt (2000).

Chapter 2
Clustering and Clusters

In this chapter, we shall show several spatial point patterns in a hypothetical area of a square 10 km on each side to understand what "clustering" or "a cluster" means and to get a basic idea of how to approach detection of *clustering* or *clusters*.

2.1 Spatial Pattern

Figure 2.1 shows a *random pattern* of spatial locations of 100 cases within a square where the spatial location of each case is completely independent of the spatial location of every other case. This random pattern is also called *complete spatial*

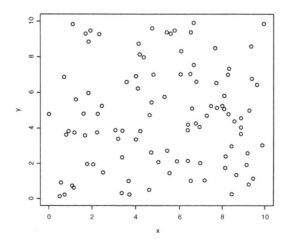

Fig. 2.1 A *random* pattern of spatial locations of 100 cases.

T. Tango, *Statistical Methods for Disease Clustering,*
Statistics for Biology and Health, DOI 10.1007/978-1-4419-1572-6_2,
© Springer Science+Business Media, LLC 2010

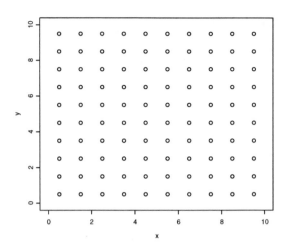

Fig. 2.2 A *completely regular* pattern of spatial locations of 100 cases.

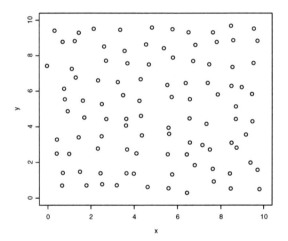

Fig. 2.3 A *regular* pattern of spatial locations of 100 cases.

randomness in the literature and is widely used as the null hypothesis of no clustering for statistical hypothesis testing. Although we can see that some points are aggregated here and there, these apparent aggregations are made up of a complete random mechanism. On the other hand, Figure 2.2 shows a completely *regular* pattern of spatial locations of 100 cases within a square where every case is the same distance from its nearest neighbor. Then, what is Figure 2.3? Is it a random pattern?

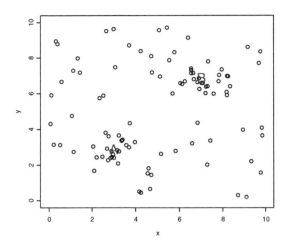

Fig. 2.4 An *aggregated* pattern (Pattern I) of spatial locations of 100 cases.

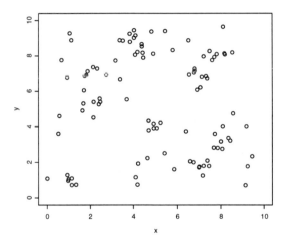

Fig. 2.5 Another *aggregated* pattern (Pattern II) of spatial locations of 100 cases.

No, it is still a *regular* pattern in the sense that cases are more spaced out than in a random pattern as in Figure 2.1. Figures 2.4 and 2.5 show two kinds of *aggregated* patterns of spatial locations, Pattern I and Pattern II, where cases are more aggregated than in a random pattern. In Figure 2.4, you may observe that cases are aggregated to a certain extent around two areas, A and B. In this situation, we call a set of aggregated cases *a cluster of cases* or *clustered cases*, and we may say that *there are two apparent clusters of cases* in this area. Some readers might be interested in the following questions:

- Is there significant clustering of cases in this area?
- How do you estimate the location of localized clusters and test their statistical significance?

Figure 2.5, on the other hand, shows that there seem to be *many small clusters of cases throughout the area*. If the disease under study is infectious, we would expect cases to be found close to each other no matter where they occur, as in Figure 2.5. Therefore, in this situation, we are not interested in localized clusters but in the question

- Is there significant clustering of cases in this area?

Before considering these questions, I would like to briefly introduce statistical models of the *spatial point process* that generates spatial point patterns.

2.2 Spatial Point Process

2.2.1 Homogeneous Poisson Process

A spatial point process describes a probabilistic model where each random variable represents the location of an event in space. In particular, a stationary and isotropic *homogeneous Poisson process* is very important and is defined by the following criteria (for example, see Diggle, 2003; Waller and Gotway, 2004, Section 5.2):

1. *Stationarity* requires that a process be invariant to translation within space.
2. *Isotropy* requires that a process be invariant to rotation about the origin.
3. The number of events occurring within an area A is a random variable following a Poisson distribution with mean $\lambda \mid A \mid$, where λ is called *intensity* and $\mid A \mid$ denotes the area of A.
4. Given the total number of events n occurring within an area A, the n events represent an independent random sample of n *locations*, each event uniformly distributed over the area.

Both stationarity and isotropy mean that the relationship between two events depends only on the distance between them. The intensity λ of the process introduced in criterion 3 means the *average number of points per unit area*; i.e., it is *estimated* by

$$\hat{\lambda} = \frac{\text{the number of events in A}}{\mid A \mid} \tag{2.1}$$

where the intensity is assumed to be constant at all locations and thus the process is called *homogeneous*. It should be noted that the "hat" over the parameter, λ here, defines an *estimate* throughout the book. Criteria 3 and 4 indicate that the numbers of events in disjoint regions are statistically independent, which is an important property for the analysis of regional count data. Finally, it should be noted that the definition above describes the statistical model for *complete spatial randomness*. The intensity is also called the *first-order* measure of a spatial point process since it describes the *mean* of the process. More useful for evaluating clustering in space is one of the *second-order* measures related to the *variance* of the process, called Ripley's K-function (Ripley, 1976, 1977), which is defined as

$$K(s) = \frac{E[\text{Number of further events within distance } s \text{ of an arbitrary event}]}{\lambda}$$

(2.2)

Under the null hypothesis of no clustering or a stationary and isotropic homogeneous Poisson process, the expected number of events within distance s of an arbitrary event is $\lambda \pi s^2$. Therefore, if there is clustering, then we expect an excess of events at short distance; i.e., $K(s) > \pi s^2$ for small s. If the boundary of the area A is sufficiently far away from all the points, then the K-function is usually calculated as

$$\hat{K}(s) = \frac{|A|}{n^2} \sum_{i=1}^{n} \sum_{j=1}^{n} I(d_{ij} \leq s)$$

where d_{ij} denotes the Euclidean distance between events i and j and $I(.)$ is the indicator function. However, in this book, we shall use the definition

$$\hat{K}(s) = \frac{|A|}{n(n-1)} \sum_{i=1}^{n} \sum_{j=1, j \neq i}^{n} I(d_{ij} \leq s)$$

(2.3)

which gives an *unbiased* estimator of the K-function (Diggle and Chetwynd, 1991). In the study of spatial point patterns generated by a homogeneous Poisson process, investigators usually have to observe the spatial pattern only in a limited area, but their major purpose is the estimation of the nature and second-order properties of the spatial patterns such as the locations of trees in a forest and cell nuclei in a microscopic tissue section rather than the clustering of events for small s. Therefore, the formula (2.3) is not appropriate for that purpose because it would not include events occurring outside the area A for s larger than the distance of an event to the nearest boundary or edge. As a method to cope with this problem, the *edge-corrected* estimator

$$\hat{K}(s) = \frac{|A|}{n(n-1)} \sum_{i=1}^{n} \sum_{j=1, j \neq i}^{n} w_{ij} I(d_{ij} \leq s)$$

(2.4)

is usually used, where w_{ij} is defined as the reciprocal of the proportion of the circumference of the circle centered at an event i with radius d_{ij} that lies within A. In other words, w_{ij} is the reciprocal of the conditional probability that an event j falls within the study region given that its distance to the event i is d_{ij}.

In the study of disease clustering, on the other hand, we are generally not interested in data outside the study area. Therefore, the K-function estimated without the edge-correction term is enough. In this book, we introduce several tests for disease clustering based on the K-function with the edge-correction term. However, when applying these methods, we have only to draw some *larger* boundary of the study region A that makes the difference between the K-function with and without the edge-correction term negligible.

2.2.2 Inhomogeneous Poisson Process

However, it is unnatural to assume a homogeneous Poisson process for examining disease clustering because the intensity strongly depends on the density of the population at risk. Therefore, we have to introduce an *inhomogeneous Poisson process* with a spatially varying intensity $\lambda(z)$ (at location z), defined as:

1. The number of events occurring within a region $D \subset A$ is a random variable following a Poisson distribution with mean $\int_D \lambda(x)dz$.
2. Given the total number of events n occurring within the study area A, the n events represent an independent random sample of n *locations* with the probability of sampling a particular point z proportional to $\lambda(z)$.

where the intensity is at least a function of the population density. However, generally the population density is not known or is difficult to compute on a local scale. Therefore, it is not practical to apply an inhomogeneous Poisson process directly to individual point data for examining disease clustering and instead we have to devise some method of escaping this difficulty.

2.3 Back to the Questions

Let us assume that the spatial distribution of the population at risk in our hypothetical area is as shown in Figure 2.6, indicating that there are two large clusters of populations at the locations similar to those of the clustered cases shown in Figure 2.4. Therefore, two apparent clusters of cases in *Pattern I* might just be due to the fact that these two areas A and B are densely populated areas. So, the problem here, based on these two types of data, the case locations and the population (or control) locations, is what kind of approach we can take to testing the null hypothesis H_0 of no clustering against the alternative hypothesis H_1:

H_0 : there is no clustering of cases in this area

H_1 : there is clustering of cases in this area

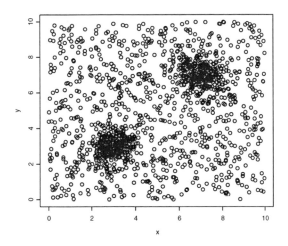

Fig. 2.6 Spatial locations of the population at risk (1500 residents).

2.4 Approaches Using Regional Count Data

If this area is partitioned into several *administrative regions* such as census tracts and block groups, an easy-to-understand and naive approach is to *count* the number of cases for each region and compare a set of *counts observed* with the corresponding set of *counts expected under the null hypothesis*. Then, let us suppose that this hypothetical area is partitioned into 25 regions or squares with each side 2 km, shown in Figure 2.7, and examine the two patterns of locations of cases above.

Example 1. Pattern I

The points A and B in Figure 2.4 are located in the regions No.7 and No. 19, respectively. Then, the observed number of cases $O_i, i = 1, ..., 25$ and the population at risk $\xi_i, i = 1, ..., 25$ per region are shown in Figure 2.8 and Figure 2.9, respectively. You can see that two regions, No.7 and No.19, have a large number of cases and large population at risk compared with other regions. So, to see if these two regions have higher rates than other regions, let us compute the observed proportion or rate per region (Figure 2.10). However, we cannot observe any high rates because the average rate is 0.064. An alternative way to look at the peculiarity of each region is to use the ratio of the *observed* (O) to the *expected* (E) number of cases, called the O/E ratio or *standardized mortality (incidence) ratio* (SMR) . The SMR in region i is defined as

$$SMR_i = \frac{O_i}{E_i} \qquad (2.5)$$

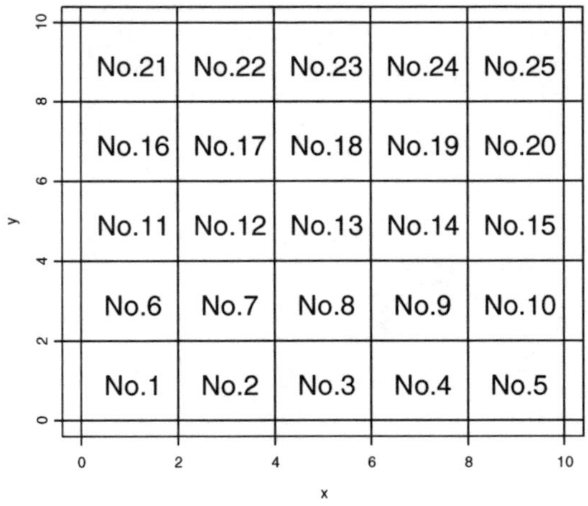

Fig. 2.7 Locations of 25 squares with each side 2 km.

where the expected number of cases E_i is calculated under the null hypothesis of no clustering. Although SMR usually refers to mortality rather than incidence, the term SMR is widely used for both mortality and morbidity, including incidence. Therefore, we shall here use the term SMR irrespective of mortality or incidence. To calculate the number of cases expected in each of 25 regions, we can apply the property of the inhomogeneous Poisson process that tells us that the number of events observed in disjoint regions still follows an independent Poisson distribution where the expected number of events in region D is proportional to $\int_D \lambda(\boldsymbol{x})d\boldsymbol{x}$. Namely, if the null hypothesis is true, the expected number of cases is proportional to the population at risk. Given the total number of cases $n = O_1 + \cdots + O_{25}$, the expected number of cases is obtained by

$$E_i = n \times \text{the ratio of the } i\text{th region's population to the total population}$$

$$= n \times \frac{\xi_i}{\sum_{j=1}^{25} \xi_j} \tag{2.6}$$

In this case, we have the following equality among the E_i's:

$$\sum_{i=1}^{25} E_i = n \tag{2.7}$$

Figure 2.11 shows SMR values for each region. SMR values greater than 1.0 indicate more cases observed than expected. The SMRs in regions No.7 and No.19 are 1.2 and 1.1, respectively, larger than 1.0 but not so large. Let us go back to the

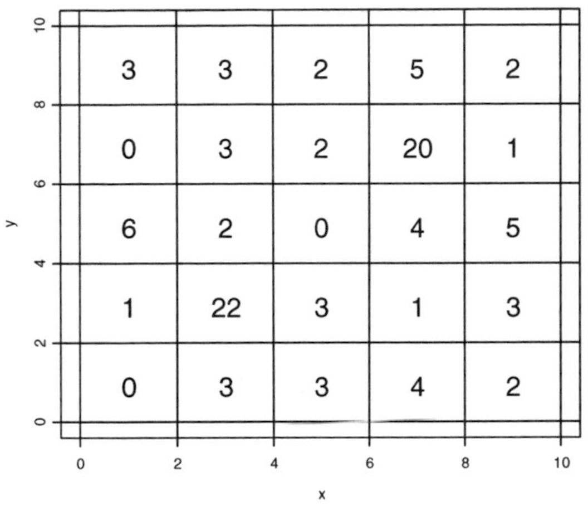

Fig. 2.8 The observed number of cases in each of 25 squares.

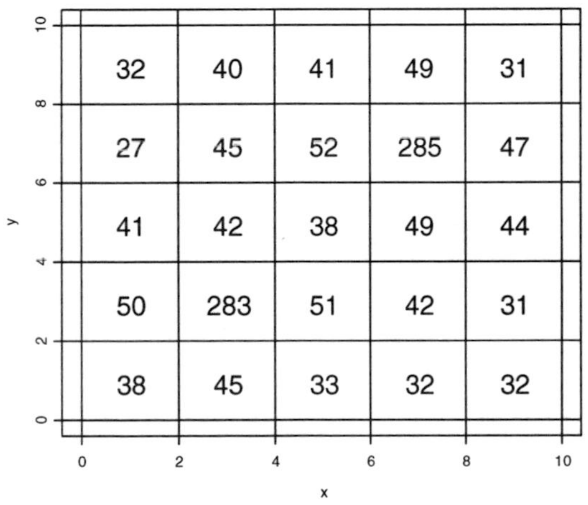

Fig. 2.9 Population at risk in each of 25 squares.

problem of testing the null hypothesis H_0 of no clustering. If we observe a number of independent cases in each region in the study area, these data can usually be analyzed by comparing the frequency distribution of counts with a Poisson distribution. If the observed number of cases O_i in region i follows independent Poisson random variables with the expected value E_i and variance E_i, then the standardized residual is given by the Z-value

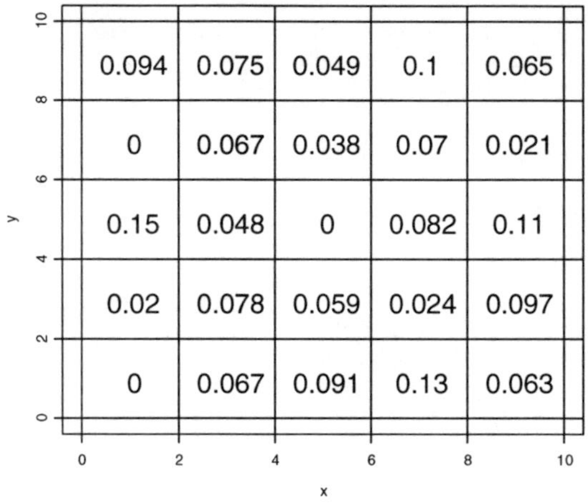
0.094 0.075 0.049 0.1 0.065
0 0.067 0.038 0.07 0.021
0.15 0.048 0 0.082 0.11
0.02 0.078 0.059 0.024 0.097
0 0.067 0.091 0.13 0.063
y
0 2 4 6 8 10
x
0 2 4 6 8 10

Fig. 2.10 Observed proportions of cases in each of 25 squares.

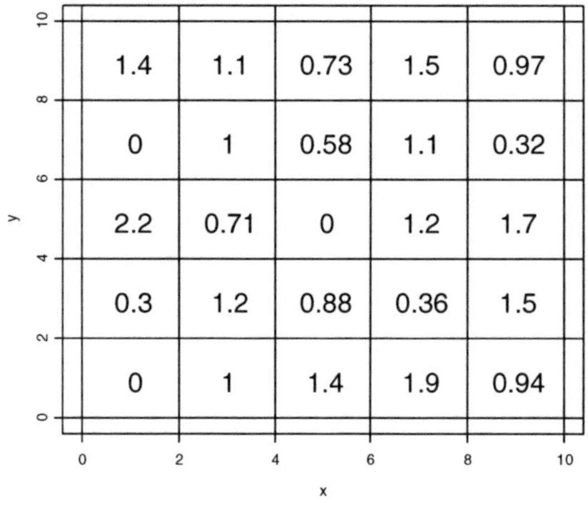
1.4 1.1 0.73 1.5 0.97
0 1 0.58 1.1 0.32
2.2 0.71 0 1.2 1.7
0.3 1.2 0.88 0.36 1.5
0 1 1.4 1.9 0.94
y
0 2 4 6 8 10
x
0 2 4 6 8 10

Fig. 2.11 Standardized mortality ratio in each of 25 squares.

$$Z_i = \frac{O_i - E_i}{\sqrt{E_i}} \tag{2.8}$$

which has approximately a standard Normal distribution $N(0,1)$ with mean zero and variance 1. Z-values larger than 2.0 or less than -2.0, say, suggest outlying high or low values. Figure 2.12 shows the individual Z-value, indicating that neither region No.7 with $Z = 0.72$ nor No.19 with $Z = 0.23$ are outlying. It should be noted

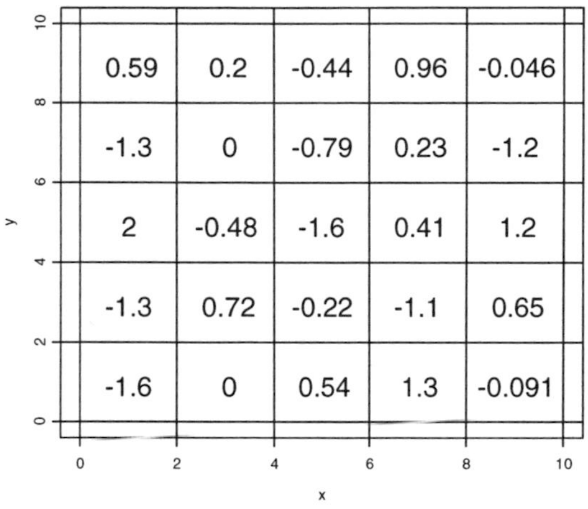

0.59	0.2	-0.44	0.96	-0.046
-1.3	0	-0.79	0.23	-1.2
2	-0.48	-1.6	0.41	1.2
-1.3	0.72	-0.22	-1.1	0.65
-1.6	0	0.54	1.3	-0.091

Fig. 2.12 Z-value in each of 25 squares.

that $(Z_1, ..., Z_{25})$ are not mutually independent because we have the equality (2.7) among the E_i's. Then, to test the null hypothesis H_0 of no clustering, we *might* use the well-known *chi-squared test statistic* X^2

$$X^2 = \sum_{i=1}^{25} Z_i^2 = \sum_{i=1}^{25} \frac{(O_i - E_i)^2}{E_i} \tag{2.9}$$

which follows an *approximately* chi-squared distribution with $24(= 25 - 1)$ degrees of freedom due to the equality (2.7) under the null hypothesis. From the Z-values in Figure 2.12, we have

$$X^2 = (-1.6)^2 + 0 + 0.54^2 + \cdots + 0.96^2 + (-0.046)^2 = 21.97$$

Then the p-value is calculated as

$$\Pr\{\chi_{24}^2 \geq 21.97\} = 0.581$$

where χ_{24}^2 denotes the random variable with a chi-squared distribution with 24 degrees of freedom (Figure 2.13). Therefore, we do not have sufficient evidence to reject the null hypothesis H_0 of no clustering at significance level 0.05.

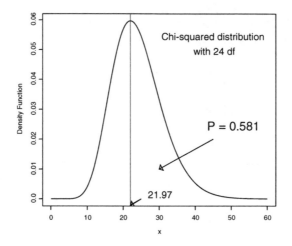

Fig. 2.13 Chi-squared distribution with 24 degrees of freedom.

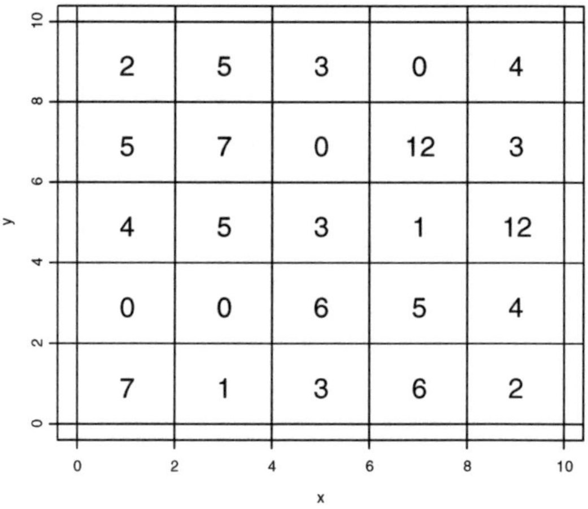

2	5	3	0	4
5	7	0	12	3
4	5	3	1	12
0	0	6	5	4
7	1	3	6	2

Fig. 2.14 Number of cases in each of 25 squares for data shown in Figure 2.5.

Example 2. Pattern II

Next, let us examine data shown in Figure 2.5 whose observed number of cases, SMRs, and Z-values in each region are shown in Figures 2.14, 2.15, and 2.16, respectively. It should be noted especially that there are *six regions* whose Z-values are larger than 2.0 or less than -2.0, namely, there are many regions with a large value of $|Z|$ indicating a typical phenomenon for Pattern II, in which cases are found close to each other throughout the area. In this case, we readily expect a large X^2, and actually we have

$$X^2 = 2.8^2 + (-1.2)^2 + \cdots + (-1.8)^2 + 1.3^2 = 100.5$$

and the p-value is

$$\Pr\{\chi^2_{24} \geq 100.5\} = 2.5 \times 10^{-11}$$

suggesting a highly significant result.

So far, we have considered what clusters and clustering mean and used a chi-squared test as an approach to test the null hypothesis H_0 of no clustering. However, there naturally arise the following questions:

- Is the use of the chi-squared distribution on the test statistic X^2 appropriate when there are several cells with zero counts or small counts?
- Is the chi-squared test appropriate in the sense that it has a reasonably good power to detect an alternative hypothesis H_1?

The first question is not so simple to answer exactly because the property that X^2 follows the chi-squared distribution with 24 degrees of freedom under H_0 is based on a *large sample approximation*. Then, the problem is, how large? However, there are some guidelines on how large the frequencies need to be for the method to be valid. The guidelines cited from Altman (1991) are that 80% of the cells (regions) should have *expected frequencies*, E_i, greater than 5, and all cells (regions) should have expected frequencies greater than 1. Notice that the observed frequencies are not involved here, only the expected frequencies. If these conditions are not met, it will be safe to employ *Monte Carlo hypothesis testing*, which will be described in Section 2.6. Figure 2.17 shows the expected number of cases in each of 25 squares for data with total number of cases $n = 100$ and population at risk as shown in Figure 2.9. In this case, although all the regions have an expected number of cases greater than 1, only two regions (8%), No. 7 and No. 19, have an expected number of cases greater than 5, indicating that the use of the chi-squared distribution with 24 degrees of freedom is doubtful. In epidemiological studies associated with disease clustering, some rare diseases are often the target of the study and the total number of cases available for study is not so large. We often encounter a similar situation in which there is a small expected number of cases in many administrative regions, partly due to the heterogeneity of the population at risk.

The second question is more important. As you can see from the form of the chi-squared test statistic (2.9), it measures *any* deviation from expectation and takes no account of spatial patterns among regions. In other words, the chi-squared test statistic is a location-invariant test statistic, that is, even if we were to randomly reassign the counts to different regions, the value of X^2 would remain the same. This is quite an undesirable property of the test statistic for detecting disease clustering and *localized disease clusters*. For example, we show three patterns of observed Z-values in each of 25 regions in Figure 2.18. When you look at these three patterns,

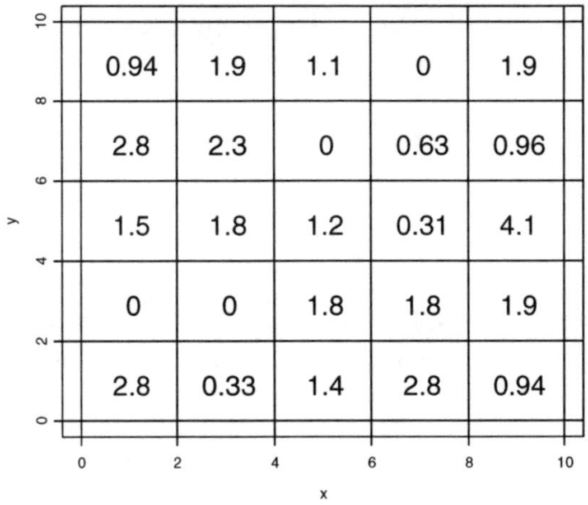

Fig. 2.15 Standardized mortality ratio in each of 25 squares for data shown in Figure 2.5.

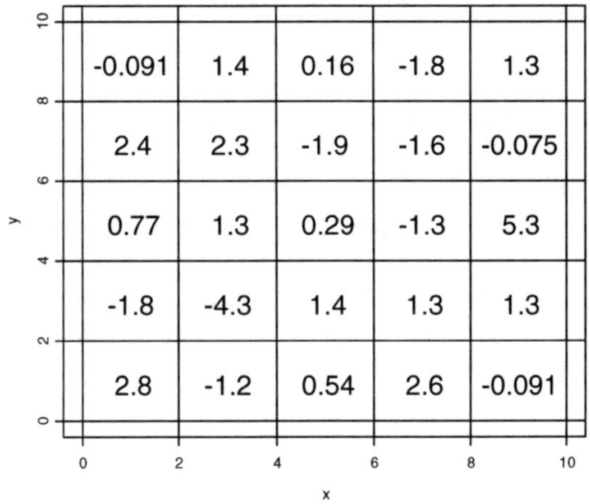

Fig. 2.16 Z-value in each of 25 squares for data shown in Figure 2.5.

it is easily understood that Pattern A has the largest *intensity of clustering* in the center of the area, Pattern B has the second largest, and Pattern C has the smallest. However, all the values of the chi-squared test statistic are the same, $X^2 = 25.0$, $P = 0.41$.

Regarding the *localized cluster*, there are two broad classes of cluster models, namely *hot-spot* clusters and *clinal* clusters (Wartenberg and Greenberg, 1990). Hot

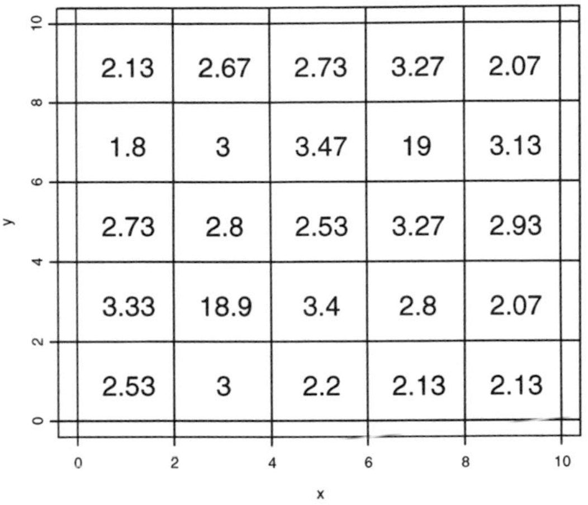

2.13	2.67	2.73	3.27	2.07
1.8	3	3.47	19	3.13
2.73	2.8	2.53	3.27	2.93
3.33	18.9	3.4	2.8	2.07
2.53	3	2.2	2.13	2.13

Fig. 2.17 Expected number of cases in each of 25 squares for data with total number of cases $n = 100$ and the population at risk shown in Figure 2.9.

spot clusters are characterized by a constant elevated disease rate in regions near the point source and a background disease rate elsewhere. Clinal clusters, on the other hand, involve a gradual decrease in disease risk as the distance from the point source increases, eventually resulting in the background rate. Figure 2.19 illustrates a plot of hypothetical relative risk surface for both hot-spot and clinal clusters. These two models are widely used in the literature of disease clustering. Therefore, the test statistic designed for detecting disease clustering must incorporate some *measure of closeness* between *observation units* or *regions* so as to have good power to detect the clustering of cases such as Pattern A in Figure 2.18 (a). For example, let a_{ij} denote some measure of closeness between regions i and j, which is usually a monotonically nonincreasing function of the distance d_{ij} between the centroids of regions i and j. One example is the *hot-spot type* measure of closeness:

$$a_{ij} = \begin{cases} 1, & d_{ij} < \lambda \ (\text{km}) \\ 0, & \text{otherwise} \end{cases} \qquad (2.10)$$

where λ denotes the *cluster size*. Then, the statistic

$$S_i = \sum_{j=1}^{m} O_j a_{ij} \qquad (2.11)$$

denotes the observed number of cases within the distance λ from region i where m denotes the number of regions in the study area. In other words, S_i denotes the observed number of cases within the *circular window* with radius λ and the center

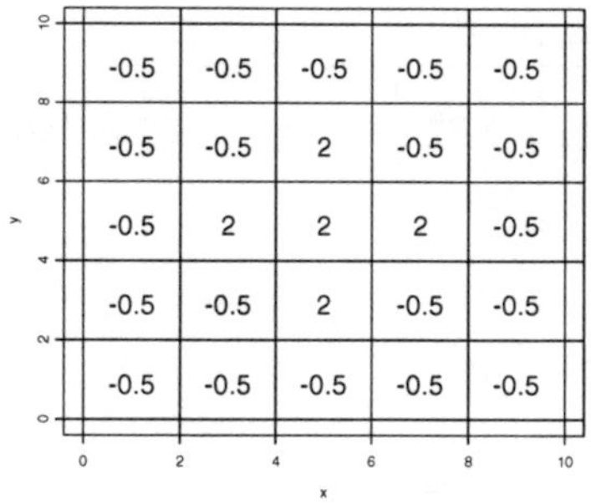

-0.5 -0.5 -0.5 -0.5 -0.5
-0.5 -0.5 2 -0.5 -0.5
-0.5 2 2 2 -0.5
-0.5 -0.5 2 -0.5 -0.5
-0.5 -0.5 -0.5 -0.5 -0.5
y
0 2 4 6 8 10
x

(a) Pattern A.

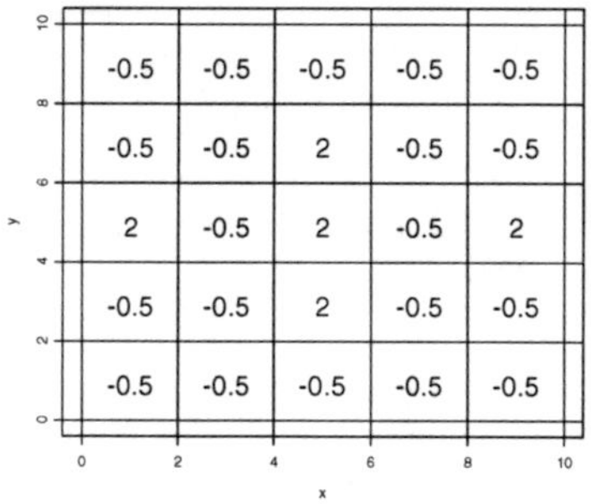

-0.5 -0.5 -0.5 -0.5 -0.5
-0.5 -0.5 2 -0.5 -0.5
2 -0.5 2 -0.5 2
-0.5 -0.5 2 -0.5 -0.5
-0.5 -0.5 -0.5 -0.5 -0.5
y
0 2 4 6 8 10
x

(b) Pattern B.

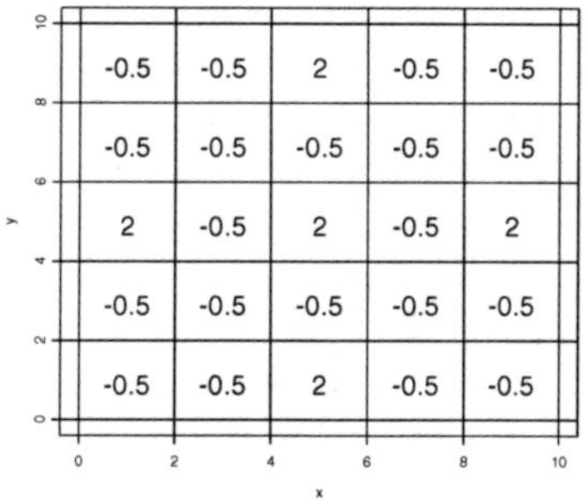

-0.5 -0.5 2 -0.5 -0.5
-0.5 -0.5 -0.5 -0.5 -0.5
2 -0.5 2 -0.5 2
-0.5 -0.5 -0.5 -0.5 -0.5
-0.5 -0.5 2 -0.5 -0.5
y
0 2 4 6 8 10
x

(c) Pattern C.

Fig. 2.18 Three spatial patterns of observed Z-values in each of 25 regions.

on the centroid of region i. We can use this type of statistic for detecting localized clusters. Kulldorff's spatial scan statistic (1997) is based on this type of statistic.

On the other hand, an example of the *clinial type* measure of closeness is

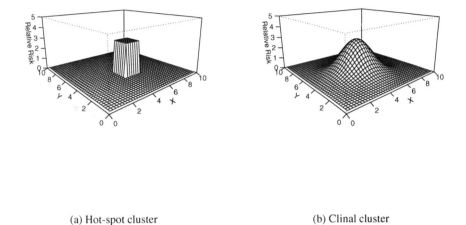

(a) Hot-spot cluster   (b) Clinal cluster

Fig. 2.19 Relative risk surfaces for a hot-spot cluster model and a clinal cluster model .

$$a_{ij} = \exp\left\{-4\left(\frac{d_{ij}}{\lambda}\right)^2\right\}. \qquad (2.12)$$

Here also λ denotes the cluster size because the value of a_{ij} is substantially zero for distances larger than λ (Figure 2.20). Then, the statistic

$$T = \sum_{i=1}^{m}\sum_{j=1}^{m} a_{ij} f(O_i, E_i) f(O_j, E_j) \qquad (2.13)$$

will be used to detect clustering throughout the area where $f(O_i, E_i)$ denotes a measure of *deviation from the expectation* in region i. Tango's (1995, 2000) index for spatial clustering is based on this type of statistic.

2.5 Approaches Using Case-Control Location Data

In general, access to individual location data is practically difficult mainly due to a confidentiality problem. If it is possible, we should select controls (noncases) randomly so that control locations can be a representative sample of the entire population in the study area. Here, let us select 100 controls from a population of 1500 as shown in Figure 2.6. Figure 2.21 shows the locations of 100 cases of Pattern I

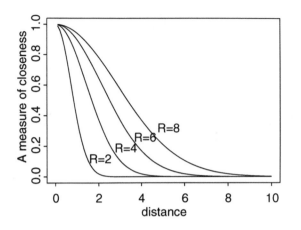

Fig. 2.20 A measure of closeness with an exponential function in distance for the case with $\lambda = 2, 4, 6, 8$ (equation (2.12)).

and 100 controls, in which two spatial patterns are very similar. On the other hand, Figure 2.22 shows spatial locations of 100 cases of Pattern II and 100 controls, in which two spatial patterns seem to be quite different. So, the problem here is how to approach testing the null hypothesis H_0 of no clustering against the alternative hypothesis H_1. In a similar way to the approach for regional count data described in the previous section, we shall define similar measures of closeness between two locations. Let a_{ij} defined in (2.10) denote here a measure of closeness between two point locations i and j. Then, a simple but natural idea would be to *count the observed number of cases within a circular window with radius λ imposed on each case*. This statistic is expressed as

$$S_i = \sum_{j=1}^{m} \delta_j a_{ij} \qquad (2.14)$$

where m denotes the total number of cases and controls and

$$\delta_i = \begin{cases} 1, & \text{if } i \text{ is a case} \\ 0, & \text{if } i \text{ is a control} \end{cases} \qquad (2.15)$$

If we are interested in detecting *localized clusters*, then we can repeat counting S_i by changing the radius and search for the optimal window or *the most likely candidate for the localized cluster*. On the other hand, if we are interested in detecting whether there is clustering throughout the area, we compute the sum, over all cases, of S_i, and the test statistic will be

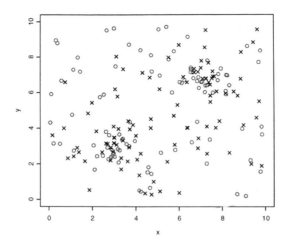

Fig. 2.21 Locations of 100 cases (○) shown in Figure 2.4 and 100 controls (×).

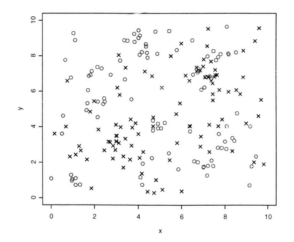

Fig. 2.22 Locations of 100 cases (○) shown in Figure 2.5 and 100 controls (×).

$$S = \sum_{i=1}^{m} \sum_{j=1}^{m} \delta_i \delta_j a_{ij} \tag{2.16}$$

Regarding the distance or the radius λ, we can consider two kinds of measures, the ordinary *Euclidean distance* and k *NN (nearest neighbors)*. Cuzick and Edwards' test (1990) for disease clustering is an example of this type with k NN.

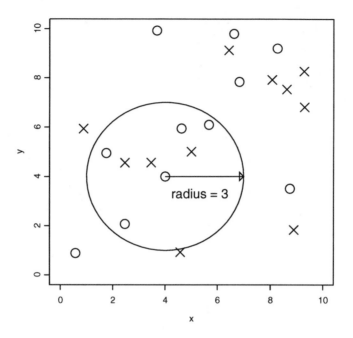

Fig. 2.23 Fictitious locations of cases ($\circ$) and controls ($\times$) illustrating the computation of the observed number of cases within distance $d = 3$ of a case located at $(4,4)$.

Figure 2.23 shows a fictitious example of locations of case-control data illustrating the computation of the observed number of cases within Euclidean distance $d = 3$ of a case located at $(4,4)$. In this example, there are a further four cases within the circular window. Figure 2.24, on the other hand, shows the same case-control locations as Figure 2.23, illustrating the computation of the observed number of cases within $k = 7$ nearest neighbors of a case located at $(4,4)$. In this example, 1NN=control, 2NN=control, 3NN=control, 4NN=case, 5NN=case, 6NN=case and 7NN=case. Therefore, there are a further four cases within this circular window also. If we apply a_{ij} defined in (2.12) to case-control location data, Tango's (2007) test can be derived.

To test the null hypothesis H_0 of no clustering, we need to compare these quantities with their expected values under the null hypothesis H_0, which usually involves complex computation. In such a case, we can rely on Monte Carlo hypothesis testing, to be described in the next section.

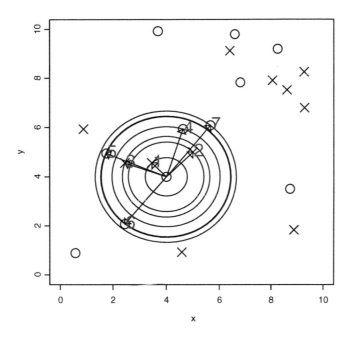

Fig. 2.24 The same locations of cases (○) and controls (×) shown in Figure 2.23 illustrating the computation of the observed number of cases within $k = 7$ nearest neighbors of a case located at $(4,4)$.

2.6 Monte Carlo Hypothesis Testing

For any statistical hypothesis test, we need the *null distribution* or the distribution of the test statistic under the null hypothesis. Some of the well-known tests such as the *Student t test* for the equality of two means and *F test* for the equality of two variances are based on the *exact null distributions, t distribution,* and *F distribution*, respectively, derived theoretically under some assumptions on the data. The null distributions for many other tests are derived by *asymptotic arguments*. However, there are many situations where the usual asymptotic distribution may be inappropriate and inaccurate, as we have already discussed regarding the validity of the chi-square distribution for the *chi-squared test statistic* (2.9) in Section 2.4. Furthermore, there are situations where it is hard to derive the null distribution even by asymptotic arguments, especially in the spatial analysis of data. In this case, Monte Carlo simulation-based hypothesis testing, called *Monte Carlo hypothesis testing* (Dwass, 1957), plays an important role. In Monte Carlo hypothesis testing,

1. First, we calculate the observed value T_{obs} of the test statistic based on the observed data as usual.
2. Second, we calculate the same statistic for a large number (say, N_{rep}) of data sets simulated independently under the null hypothesis of no clustering and let these values be $\{T_1, T_2, \ldots, T_{N_{\text{rep}}}\}$.
3. The proportion of test statistic values based on simulated data exceeding the observed value of the test statistic provides a Monte Carlo estimate of the upper-tail p value. That is, if T_{obs} ranks the R largest among $N_{\text{rep}} + 1$ values of T's, then the simulated upper tail p-value is given by

$$\text{Simulated } p\text{-value} = \frac{R}{N_{\text{rep}} + 1} \qquad (2.17)$$

or equivalently

$$\text{Simulated } p\text{-value} = \frac{1 + \sum_{v=1}^{N_{\text{rep}}} I(T_v \geq T_{\text{obs}})}{N_{\text{rep}} + 1} \qquad (2.18)$$

where $I(.)$ is the indicator function. The lower-tail p-value is calculated similarly.

Needless to say, Monte Carlo simulated p-values are not calculated uniquely due to randomly simulated data. In other words, another independent set of N_{rep} realizations will result in a slightly different p-value. However, the larger the number of repetitions N_{rep}, the more stable the resulting p-values. Usually, the value of N_{rep} is set as 999, 9999, and so on.

2.7 Spatial Autocorrelation

A positive *spatial autocorrelation* implies that *pairs of observations taken nearby are more similar than those taken far apart*, which will be a key issue in statistical modeling of spatial epidemiology. For example, when we are performing spatial regression to determine what covariate, such as age, mean income, educational levels, or ethnic origin, contributes to a higher risk for a disease under study, it is critical to adjust for the spatial autocorrelation in the data. Otherwise, the risk will be overestimated, with biased p-values that are too small, providing "statistically significant" results when none exist. Here, the null hypothesis should be that there is spatial autocorrelation, and the alternative hypothesis should be that there are both spatial autocorrelation and geographical differences in the risk of the disease. See also Section 3.5 for hierarchical Bayesian regression models. Furthermore, it should be noted that there are two famous global indices of spatial autocorrelation, Moran's I and Geary's c (see Section 5.3).

On the other hand, if we are interested in detecting disease clustering or disease clusters, we should not adjust for the spatial autocorrelation since we are interested in detecting clusters due to such autocorrelation, and if they are adjusted away, important clusters might go undetected. Here, the null hypothesis is that cases are geographically randomly distributed (adjusted for population density, etc.), and the alternative hypothesis is that there is some clustering either due to differences in underlying risk factors or spatial autocorrelation.

Chapter 3
Disease Mapping: Visualization of Spatial Clustering

Disease mapping is the most basic way of visualizing the spatial distribution of the disease of interest in a defined area.

Example 1: Snow's Map

Figure 3.1 shows the map of addresses of those who died of cholera and locations of water supply pumps used in the study by John Snow (1854) on the cholera epidemics

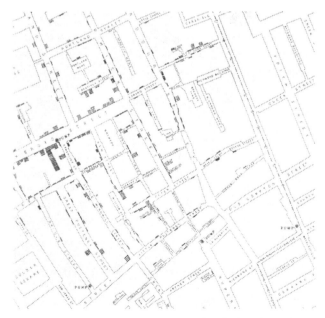

Fig. 3.1 Map of addresses of deaths from cholera related to the locations of water supply pumps at Golden Square.

T. Tango, *Statistical Methods for Disease Clustering*,
Statistics for Biology and Health, DOI 10.1007/978-1-4419-1572-6_3,
© Springer Science+Business Media, LLC 2010

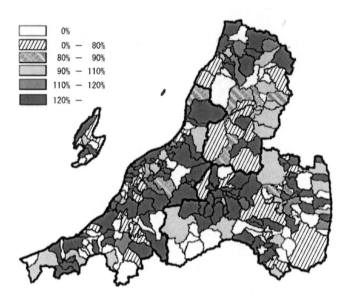

Fig. 3.2 Choropleth map of standardized mortality ratios (SMRs) of gallbladder cancer (male) in three adjacent prefectures, Niigata, Fukushima, and Yamagata, consisting of 246 villages, towns, and cities in Japan for the years 1996–2000, based on the age-specific mortality rates from the 1985 national census population.

spread around the Golden Square area in London during the middle of the nineteenth century. This was the first and most famous disease map used in an epidemiological study, which evidently suggested a significant clustering of cholera victims around water supply pumps.

Example 2

Figure 3.2 shows an example of a choropleth map of standardized mortality ratios (SMRs) of gallbladder cancer (male) in three adjacent prefectures, Niigata, Fukushima, and Yamagata, consisting of 246 villages, towns, and cities in Japan for the years 1996–2000, based on the age-specific mortality rates from the 1985 national census population. The total observed number of deaths for the five years was 665.

In a study of geographical variations of disease risk, the locations of cases are usually residential addresses such as zip code or postal code unit. If such individual addresses are available, it will be easy to plot the locations of cases on the local *white map* or using some Cartesian coordinates. John Snow's map of the Golden Square cholera epidemic (Figure 3.1) shows the usefulness of the disease mapping method. However, due to confidentiality requirements in medical studies, it is not often possible to obtain individual-level addresses and it is instead possible to obtain only as aggregate counts for each of the defined regions. In the case of aggregate count data, choropleth maps are the most common type of map for visualizing the spatial distribution of disease in each of the defined regions using such health indices as prevalence, incidence rate and mortality rate. Choropleth maps usually use different color or pattern combinations to depict different levels of disease risk associated with each region. These regions are small areas usually defined for administrative purposes, such as census tracts, counties, electoral wards, villages and towns, and cities. Figure 3.2 indicates an example of a choropleth map of standardized mortality ratios of gallbladder cancer (male), in which the dark (red in the e-book) regions have the highest ratios (120% <) of gallbladder cancer and regions with white color have the lowest ratios (0%); i.e., the observed number of deaths is zero.

In this chapter, we shall introduce basic ideas of disease mapping and a range of mapping methods, including Bayesian models, which are useful tools for visualizing regional variation of disease risk or regional clustering and/or clusters. Together with the statistical tests for disease clustering described in Chapters 4–9, we would like to recommend the joint use of *smoothed* disease maps estimated by Bayesian models based on the Markov chain Monte Carlo technique. This is because interpretation of test results could be clear and/or easy compared with the smoothed disease maps. However, as the details of these methods fall beyond the scope of this text, see Gilks, Richardson and Spiegelhalter (1996), Lawson, Brown, and Rodeiro (2003), and Lawson (2008), for example.

3.1 Standardization

When we examine a spatial variation of some mortality rate among regions, it is quite important to eliminate the effects of known confounding factors. *Age* is the most important confounding factor since there is an increasing mortality (incidence) of disease with age, especially at ages greater than 40 years. For example, regions with more elderly populations will have higher mortality rates than those with younger populations. We are not interested in the difference in rates entirely due to the different age distributions; rather we are interested in the difference in rates adjusted for these confounding factors. To find this, we can apply the so-called method of *standardization*. There are two types of standardization: *direct standardization* and *indirect standardization*. In either case, a common *standard population* must be chosen to adjust rates to reflect the age distribution within the standard population. A typical selection for standard populations could be the population from a national census that includes the study population. Then, the difference in these standardizations can be stated as follows:

- *Direct standardization* utilizes observed age-specific rates within the study population *directly* to estimate the *expected number of cases in the standard population*.

- *Indirect standardization* utilizes the age-specific rates within the standard population (*indirectly*) to estimate the *expected number of cases in the study population*.

Suppose we have m regions and K age groups, and let n_{ik} and ξ_{ik} denote the number of cases and the number of people at risk in the kth age group and the ith region for the study population, respectively, where $i = 1, ..., m$ and $k = 1, ..., K$. Then, define $r_{ik} = n_{ik}/\xi_{ik}$ to be the observed mortality rate in the kth age group and the ith region. Similarly, let $n_{ik}^{(s)}, \xi_{ik}^{(s)}$, and $r_{ik}^{(s)}$ denote the number of cases, number of people at risk, and the observed mortality rate for the standard population. Then, direct standardization estimates $D_{+k}^{(s)}$, the number of cases expected in the standard population within the kth age group, as

$$D_{ik} = r_{ik} * \xi_{+k}^{(s)} = \frac{n_{ik}}{\xi_{ik}} \xi_{+k}^{(s)} \qquad (3.1)$$

Then, the overall mortality rate expected in the standard population, called the DSR (directly standardized mortality rate), is defined as

$$DSR_i = \frac{\sum_{k=1}^{K} D_{ik}}{\xi_{++}^{(s)}} = \sum_{k=1}^{K} \frac{\xi_{+k}^{(s)}}{\xi_{++}^{(s)}} \frac{n_{ik}}{\xi_{ik}} \qquad (3.2)$$

Figure 3.3 shows a choropleth map of the DSR of gallbladder cancer (male, per 100,000) in three adjacent prefectures, Niigata, Fukushima, and Yamagata, consisting of 246 villages, towns, and cities in Japan (1996–2000), using the 1985 national census to represent the standard population. On the other hand, indirect standardization computes the expected number of cases in the study population, which is given by

$$e_i = \sum_{k=1}^{K} \frac{n_{ik}^{(s)}}{\xi_{ik}^{(s)}} \xi_{ik}. \qquad (3.3)$$

The most common health index based on the expected number of cases in the study population is the so-called observed/expected ratio or standardized mortality ratio (SMR), which is given by

$$SMR_i = \frac{n_i}{e_i}, \ (n_i := n_{i+}) \qquad (3.4)$$

The region with SMR greater than 1.0 indicates more cases observed in the study population than expected from the age-specific mortality rates in the standard population. The SMR values are often reported as a percentage by multiplying the ratio by 100. Using the SMRs and the crude mortality rate in the standard population provides the ISR (indirectly standardized mortality rate) :

$$ISR_i = SMR_i \frac{n_{++}^{(s)}}{\xi_{++}^{(s)}} \qquad (3.5)$$

However, ISR is not often used in epidemiological literature compared with SMR since ISR is proportional to SMR and the interpretation of SMR is more understandable. Figure 3.4 shows a choropleth map of the SMR of gallbladder cancer (male) similar to the map shown in Figure 3.2. However, this map is based on the age-specific mortality rates from the standard population consisting of three prefectures combined, not of the 1985 census population in Japan. To examine the existence of spatial clustering or localized spatial clusters within the defined study area, the entire study area should be used as a standard population.

As shown in Figures 3.2 and 3.4, SMRs are frequently used in disease maps. SMRs, however, have the undesirable property that they can be greatly affected by relatively small changes in expected value, especially when the expected value is small. In general, the expected number of cases is proportional to the population size. Therefore, there are more variations of SMRs in small cities than in large cities. Figure 3.5 shows the variations of SMRs against the log-transformed population size for the choropleth map of the SMR of gallbladder cancer in males (Figure 3.4) This figure clearly indicates that the variation of SMR is inversely proportional to the population or the expected number of cases. Therefore, it would be very dangerous for public health officials to examine which region truly has the largest or lowest rates based on SMRs because the population size strongly affects the variability of SMR values. So, we have to use some sort of population-adjusted SMR. In what follows, we shall deal with the problem of spatial variation of disease risks within the framework of statistical models.

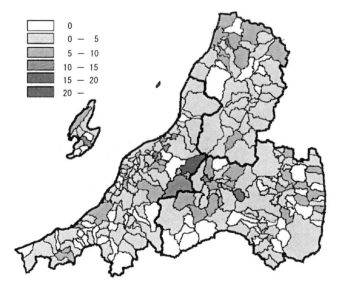

Fig. 3.3 Choropleth map of DSR of gallbladder cancer (male, per 100,000) in three adjacent prefectures, Niigata, Fukushima, and Yamagata, consisting of 246 villages, towns, and cities in Japan (1996–2000), using the 1985 national census to represent the standard population.

3.2 Basic Models for Relative Risk

Let N_i denote the random variable of the observed number of cases n_i in region $i(= 1, ..., m)$. Then we assume that the N_i are independently distributed with a Poisson distribution with the mean proportional to the expected number of cases calculated from some standard population,

$$N_i \sim \text{Poisson}(\theta_i e_i) \tag{3.6}$$

where θ_i denotes the relative risk of disease under study in region i and Poisson(μ) denotes the Poisson distribution with mean μ, and its probability distribution function is

$$\Pr\{N_i = n_i \mid \theta_i, e_i\} = f(n_i|\theta_i, e_i) = \frac{(\theta_i e_i)^{n_i} \exp(-\theta_i e_i)}{n_i!} \tag{3.7}$$

$$E(n_i) = \theta_i e_i \tag{3.8}$$

$$\text{Var}(n_i) = \theta_i e_i \tag{3.9}$$

If $\theta_1 = \cdots = \theta_m$, then we can say that there is no spatial variation of disease risk or no spatial clustering of disease. Different estimators of θ_i will be derived depending on the way of modeling $\{\theta_i\}$.

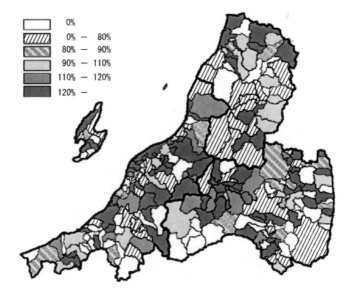

Fig. 3.4 Choropleth map of standardized mortality ratios (SMRs) of gallbladder cancer (male) in three adjacent prefectures, Niigata, Fukushima, and Yamagata, consisting of 246 villages, towns, and cities in Japan for the years 1996–2000, based on the age-specific mortality rates from the three prefectures combined.

3.3 Likelihood Models

Let us consider here the most simple model for the relative risk, where θ_i denotes a constant or *fixed-effects* parameter of the relative risk of disease under study in region i. Under the model above, the likelihood for $\boldsymbol{\theta} = (\theta_1, ..., \theta_m)^t$ is

$$L(\boldsymbol{\theta}) = \prod_{i=1}^{m} \left(\frac{(\theta_i e_i)^{n_i} \exp(-\theta_i e_i)}{n_i!} \right) \tag{3.10}$$

and then the log-likelihood is, bar a constant,

$$l(\boldsymbol{\theta}) = \log L(\boldsymbol{\theta}) = \sum_{i=1}^{m} (n_i \log(\theta_i e_i) - \theta_i e_i) \tag{3.11}$$

Then, the maximum likelihood estimator of θ_i and its variance are given by

$$\hat{\theta}_i = \frac{n_i}{e_i} \quad \text{(just the SMR)} \tag{3.12}$$

$$\text{Var}(\hat{\theta}_i) = \frac{\theta_i}{e_i} \tag{3.13}$$

The variance of the SMR is inversely proportional to e_i, indicating the variation of the SMRs shown in Figure 3.5. However, as already described earlier, the SMRs are not always an appropriate measure for disease mapping, especially when the differences in population size among regions are quite large. To cope with the drawback of the SMRs, several methods have been proposed in the literature.

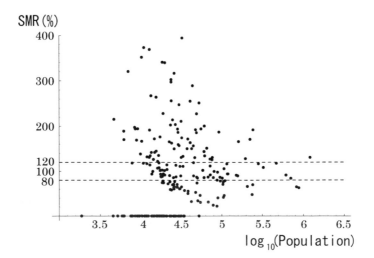

Fig. 3.5 SMRs against the log-transformed population size.

3.4 Poisson-Gamma Bayesian Models

One of the most promising methods will be a Bayesian approach, where we consider the *random-effects* relative risk θ_i with prior distribution $g(\theta \mid \boldsymbol{\eta})$ and inference is based on the mean of the posterior distribution of $\boldsymbol{\theta} = (\theta_1, ..., \theta_m)$ given the data. One of the classical prior distributions on the relative risk is a gamma distribution with hyperparameters $\boldsymbol{\eta} = (\alpha, \beta)$,

$$\theta_i \sim \text{Gamma}(\alpha, \beta) \tag{3.14}$$

where the density function is given by

$$g(\theta \mid \alpha, \beta) = \frac{\beta(\beta\theta)^{\alpha-1} \exp(-\beta\theta)}{\Gamma(\alpha)} \tag{3.15}$$

$$E(\theta) = \frac{\alpha}{\beta} \tag{3.16}$$

$$\text{Var}(\theta) = \frac{\alpha}{\beta^2} \tag{3.17}$$

This prior distribution is called a *conjugate prior* because the posterior distribution is also the same type of prior distribution. Based on Bayes' theorem, the posterior distribution of θ_i is given by

$$h(\theta_i \mid n_i, e_i, \boldsymbol{\eta}) = \frac{g(\theta_i \mid \boldsymbol{\eta}) f(n_i \mid \theta_i, e_i)}{\int_0^\infty g(\theta \mid \boldsymbol{\eta}) f(n_i \mid \theta, e_i) d\theta}$$
$$= g(\theta_i \mid n_i + \alpha, e_i + \beta) \tag{3.18}$$

Then, the Bayes estimator $\hat{\theta}_{i,B}$ is the posterior expectation

$$\hat{\theta}_{i,B} = E(\theta_i \mid e_i, d_i, \boldsymbol{\eta})$$
$$= \int_0^\infty \theta h(\theta \mid e_i, d_i, \boldsymbol{\eta}) d\theta$$
$$= \frac{\int_0^\infty \theta g(\theta \mid \boldsymbol{\eta}) f(d_i \mid \theta, e_i) d\theta}{\int_0^\infty g(\theta \mid \boldsymbol{\eta}) f(d_i \mid \theta, e_i) d\theta}$$
$$= \frac{n_i + \alpha}{e_i + \beta}$$
$$= \frac{e_i}{e_i + \beta} \frac{n_i}{e_i} + \frac{\beta}{e_i + \beta} \frac{\alpha}{\beta} \tag{3.19}$$

Namely, the Bayes estimator is a weighted average of the SMR for the region i and the global mean in the entire study area. Furthermore, we have the following property:

1. When the population size or the expected number of cases is large, the Bayes estimator tends to approach to the SMR, n_i/e_i.

2. When the population size is small, the Bayes estimator tends to be close to the overall mean, $\alpha = \beta$.

Then, the problem here is how to estimate $\boldsymbol{\eta} = (\alpha, \beta)$.

3.4.1 Empirical Bayes Estimator

(*Readers who are not interested in the estimation method can skip the corresponding details.*)

One approach is to use the maximum likelihood estimator $\hat{\boldsymbol{\eta}} = (\hat{\alpha}, \hat{\beta})$ for the *marginal distribution* of the number of cases N_i,

$$\prod_{i=1}^{m} \Pr\{N_i = n_i \mid e_i, \boldsymbol{\eta}\} = \prod_{i=1}^{m} \int_{0}^{\infty} g(\theta \mid \boldsymbol{\eta}) f(d_i \mid \theta, e_i) d\theta \qquad (3.20)$$

which is called the *marginal maximum likelihood* estimator or *empirical Bayes estimator*, in the sense that the parameters $\boldsymbol{\eta} = (\alpha, \beta)$ are estimated directly by the data. In the Poisson-gamma model above, this distribution is a negative binomial distribution,

$$\Pr\{N_i = n_i \mid e_i, \alpha, \beta\} = \frac{\Gamma(n_i + \alpha)}{\Gamma(\alpha) n_i!} \left(\frac{\beta}{e_i + \beta} \right)^{\alpha} \left(\frac{e_i}{e_i + \beta} \right)^{n_i} \qquad (3.21)$$

$$E(N_i) = \frac{e_i \alpha}{\beta} \qquad (3.22)$$

$$\text{Var}(N_i) = \frac{e_i(e_i + \beta)\alpha}{\beta^2} \qquad (3.23)$$

The moment estimator for (α, β) is given by the solutions of the equations

$$E\left\{ \sum_{i=1}^{m} \frac{1}{m} \frac{n_i}{e_i} \right\} = \frac{\alpha}{\beta} \qquad (3.24)$$

$$E\left\{ \frac{1}{m} \sum_{i=1}^{m} \left(\frac{n_i}{e_i} - \frac{\alpha}{\beta} \right)^2 \right\} = \frac{\alpha}{\beta^2} + \frac{\alpha}{\beta} \frac{1}{m} \sum_{i=1}^{m} \frac{1}{e_i} \qquad (3.25)$$

The log-likelihood is, bar a constant,

$$l(\alpha, \beta) = \log \sum_{i=1}^{m} \Pr\{n_i \mid e_i, \alpha, \beta\}$$

$$= \sum_{i=1}^{m} \sum_{s=0}^{n_i-1} \log(\alpha + s) + m\alpha \log \beta - \alpha \sum_{i=1}^{m} \log(\beta + e_i)$$

$$- \sum_{i=1}^{m} n_i \log(\beta + e_i) \qquad (3.26)$$

Then, the marginal maximum likelihood estimator for (α, β) is the solution of the equations

$$\frac{\partial l}{\partial \alpha} = \frac{\partial l}{\partial \beta} = 0$$

which is given by the Newton-Raphson iterative method

$$\begin{bmatrix} \hat{\alpha} \\ \hat{\beta} \end{bmatrix}_{(k+1)} = \begin{bmatrix} \hat{\alpha} \\ \hat{\beta} \end{bmatrix}_{(k)} + \begin{bmatrix} -\frac{\partial^2 l}{\partial \alpha^2} & -\frac{\partial^2 l}{\partial \alpha \partial \beta} \\ -\frac{\partial^2 l}{\partial \beta \partial \alpha} & -\frac{\partial^2 l}{\partial \beta^2} \end{bmatrix}_{(k)}^{-1} \begin{bmatrix} \frac{\partial l}{\partial \alpha} \\ \frac{\partial l}{\partial \beta} \end{bmatrix}_{(k)} \tag{3.27}$$

where

$$\frac{\partial l}{\partial \alpha} = m\frac{\alpha}{\beta} - \sum_{i=1}^{m} \frac{\alpha + d_i}{\beta + e_i}$$

$$\frac{\partial l}{\partial \beta} = \sum_{i=1}^{m} \sum_{s=0}^{n_i-1} \frac{1}{\alpha + s} - \sum_{i=1}^{m} \log\left(1 + \frac{e_i}{\beta}\right)$$

$$\frac{\partial^2 l}{\partial \alpha^2} = -\frac{m\alpha}{\beta^2} + \sum_{i=1}^{m} \frac{\alpha + n_i}{(\beta + e_i)^2}$$

$$\frac{\partial^2 l}{\partial \beta^2} = -\sum_{i=1}^{m} \sum_{s=0}^{n_i-1} \frac{1}{(\alpha + s)^2}$$

$$\frac{\partial^2 l}{\partial \alpha \partial \beta} = \frac{m}{\beta} - \sum_{i=1}^{m} \frac{1}{\beta + e_i}$$

Moment estimators can be used as initial values of the iteration method. Figure 3.6 shows the choropleth map of the empirical Bayes estimate of relative risk of gall-bladder cancer (male) in three adjacent prefectures, Niigata, Fukushima, and Yamagata, based on the age-specific mortality rates from the standard population consisting of the three prefectures combined. Figure 3.7 shows the variation of empirical Bayes estimates against the log-transformed population size for the choropleth map (Figure 3.6). This figure clearly indicates that the variation of empirical Bayes estimates is smaller in regions with small population size compared with the SMRs of Figure 3.5.

3.4.2 Hierarchical Full Bayes Estimator

Another approach to estimating the parameters $\boldsymbol{\eta} = (\alpha, \beta)$ is to obtain the full Bayes estimator where these parameters are assumed to be not constant but *random variables* with prior distributions. Within the framework of full Bayesian inference, these parameters are called *hyperparameters*, and their prior distributions are called *hyperprior distributions* . In the Poisson-gamma model, there is a two-level

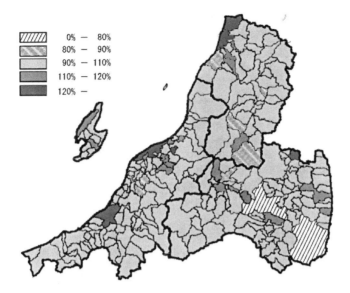

Fig. 3.6 Choropleth map of empirical Bayes estimates of relative risk of gallbladder cancer (male) in three adjacent prefectures, Niigata, Fukushima, and Yamagata, based on the age-specific mortality rates from the standard population consisting of the three prefectures combined.

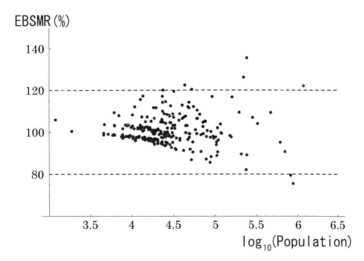

Fig. 3.7 Empirical Bayes estimates of relative risk against the log-transformed population size.

hierarchy: θ has a gamma distributin with parameters (α, β) at the first level of the hierarchy, and the α and β will have hyperpriors $h_\alpha(\cdot)$ and $h_\beta(\cdot)$, respectively, at the second level of the hierarchy. This can be expressed as

$$N_i \sim \text{Poisson}(\theta_i e_i)$$
$$\theta_i \sim \text{Gamma}(\alpha, \beta)$$
$$\alpha \sim h_\alpha$$
$$\beta \sim h_\beta$$

Regarding the selection of hyperprior distributions, *noninformative priors* are usually applied. For example, the following exponential distributions can be used for h_α and h_β:

$$\alpha \sim \text{Exponential}(\lambda), \ \lambda = 1/20$$
$$\beta \sim \text{Exponential}(\lambda), \ \lambda = 1/20$$

To execute these rather complex hierarchical Bayesian models, Markov chain Monte Carlo (MCMC) methods of posterior sampling based on computer-generated random numbers are very convenient. Such packages as WinBUGS and GeoBUGS have been widely used. See the following Website:

http://www.mrc-bsu.cam.ac.uk/bugs/

Figure 3.8 shows a choropleth map of the full Bayes estimate of relative risk (using WinBUGS) of gallbladder cancer (male) in three adjacent prefectures, Niigata, Fukushima, and Yamagata, based on the age-specific mortality rates from the standard population consisting of the three prefectures combined. We can observe that there is only a small increase in the variability of estimates compared with the map of empirical Bayes estimates.

3.5 Hierarchical Bayesian Models

3.5.1 Log-normal Model

The Poisson-gamma model is computationally convenient in the sense that the posterior distribution is also a gamma distribution. However, it is difficult to adjust for covariates and also to take the spatial autocorrelation, if any, among risks in adjacent regions into account. Therefore, in the hierarchical Bayesian models for relative risk, the log-normal model or random-effects Poisson regression model

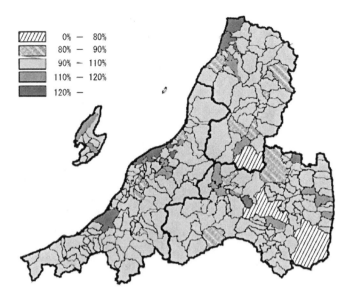

Fig. 3.8 Choropleth map of a Poisson-gamma model-based full Bayes estimate of relative risk of gallbladder cancer (male) in three adjacent prefectures, Niigata, Fukushima, and Yamagata, consisting of 246 villages, towns, and cities in Japan for the years 1996–2000, based on the age-specific mortality rates from the standard population consisting of the three prefectures combined.

$$d_i \sim \text{Poisson}(e_i \theta_i)$$
$$\log \theta_i = \mu + \varepsilon_i \qquad\qquad (3.28)$$
$$\varepsilon_i \sim N(0, \sigma_\varepsilon^2)$$

has been utilized where μ denotes an overall level of the relative risk (in log scale) and ε_i denotes the uncorrelated heterogeneity, unstructured residual, or overdispersion parameter (assuming no spatial autocorrelation). The parameters μ and σ_ε^2 will have the following hyperprior distributions:

$$\mu \sim N(0, 10^5)$$
$$1/\sigma_\varepsilon^2 \sim \text{Gamma}(0.5, 0.0005)$$

Figure 3.9 shows the choropleth map of the log-normal model-based full Bayes estimate of relative risk of gallbladder cancer (of male) in three adjacent prefectures, Niigata, Fukushima, and Yamagata, consisting of 246 villages, towns, and cities in Japan for the years 1996–2000, based on the age-specific mortality rates from the standard population consisting of the three prefectures combined. The disease map illustrated in this map is quite similar to the one obtained using the Poisson-gamma model (Figure 3.8).

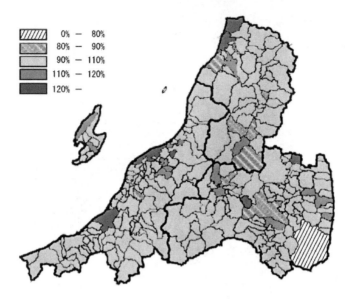

Fig. 3.9 Choropleth map of the log-normal model-based full Bayes estimate of relative risk of gall-bladder cancer (male) in three adjacent prefectures, Niigata, Fukushima, and Yamagata, consisting of 246 villages, towns, and cities in Japan for the years 1996–2000, based on the age-specific mortality rates from the standard population consisting of the three prefectures combined.

3.5.2 Conditional Autoregressive Model

The models above do not take spatial autocorrelation into account. However, we can observe spatial autocorrelation such that the relative risks among adjacent regions are quite similar to each other in many choropleth maps of diseases. Therefore it would be very natural to introduce models with spatial autocorrelation. One of the most widely used models of this type is a random-effects Poisson model allowing for overdispersion (uncorrelated heterogeneity), spatial autocorrelation, and covariate adjustments using the conditional autoregressive (CAR) model developed by Besag, York, and Mollie (1991)

$$d_i \sim \text{Poisson}(e_i\theta_i)$$
$$\log\theta_i = \mu + \beta_1 x_{1i} + \cdots + \beta_p x_{pi} + \varepsilon_i + \phi_i$$
$$(x_{1i}, ..., x_{pi}) \; : \; \text{covariates}$$
$$\varepsilon_i \sim N(0, \sigma_\varepsilon^2)$$
$$\phi_i \mid \phi_{j\neq i} \sim N\left(\bar{\phi}_i, \frac{1}{m_i}\sigma_\phi^2\right) : \quad \text{CAR model}$$
$$m_i = \text{number of regions adjacent to region } i$$
$$\bar{\phi}_i = \text{average of } \phi_j \text{ among regions adjacent to region } i$$

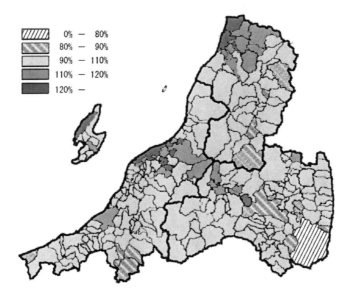

Fig. 3.10 Choropleth map of CAR model-based full Bayes estimate of relative risk of gallbladder cancer (male) in three adjacent prefectures, Niigata, Fukushima, and Yamagata, consisting of 246 villages, towns, and cities in Japan for the years 1996–2000, based on the age-specific mortality rates from the standard population consisting of the three prefectures combined.

where the following three hyperprior distributions were assumed:

$$\mu \sim \text{ improper prior}$$
$$1/\sigma_\varepsilon^2 \sim \text{Gamma}(0.5, 0.0005)$$
$$1/\sigma_\phi^2 \sim \text{Gamma}(0.5, 0.0005)$$

Figure 3.10 shows the choropleth map of the CAR model-based full Bayes estimate of relative risk of gallbladder cancer (male) in three adjacent prefectures, Niigata, Fukushima, and Yamagata, consisting of 246 villages, towns, and cities in Japan for the years 1996–2000, based on the age-specific mortality rates from the standard population consisting of the three prefectures combined. The CAR model-based Bayes estimates of relative risk indicate less variation and are smoother than the previous two Bayesian estimates.

Chapter 4

Tests for Temporal Clustering

We shall consider here the problem of detecting disease clustering in time, which is illustrated by the following two examples (Tables 4.1–4.2).

Table 4.1 $n = 35$ cases of oesophageal atresia and tracheo-oesophageal fistula over $T = 2191$ days from 1950 to 1955. Day 1 was set as 1 January 1950. (data from Knox, 1959).

No.	Interval Day number	Frequency per d days		
		$d = 100$	200	365
1	0– 99	0		
2	100–199 170	1	1	
3	200–299	0		
4	300–399 316	1	1	2
5	400–499 445, 468	2		
6	500–599	0	2	
7	600–699	0		
8	700–799	0	0	2
9	800–899	0		
10	900–999 938	1	1	
11	1000–1099 1034	1		2
12	1100–1199 1128	1	2	
13	1200–1299 1233, 1248, 1249, 1252, 1259, 1267	6		
14	1300–1399 1305, 1385, 1388, 1390	4	10	
15	1400–1499 1446, 1454, 1458, 1461, 1491	5		14
16	1500–1599 1583	1	6	
17	1600–1699 1699	1		
18	1700–1799 1702, 1787	2	3	
19	1800–1899	0		6
20	1900–1999 1924, 1974	2	2	
21	2000–2099 2049, 2051, 2067, 2075	4		
22	2100–2191 2108, 2151, 2174	3	7	9
	Total	35		

T. Tango, *Statistical Methods for Disease Clustering*,
Statistics for Biology and Health, DOI 10.1007/978-1-4419-1572-6_4,
© Springer Science+Business Media, LLC 2010

Table 4.2 Frequency of trisomy among karyotyped spontaneous abortions of pregnancies by calendar month of the last menstrual period from July 1975 to June 1977 in three New York hospitals (data from Tango, 1984).

year	month	Frequency	
		per month	per two month
1975	7	0	
	8	4	4
	9	1	
	10	2	3
	11	1	
	12	3	4
1976	1	1	
	2	3	4
	3	2	
	4	2	4
	5	3	
	6	4	7
	7	1	
	8	1	2
	9	1	
	10	2	3
	11	4	
	12	7	11
1977	1	7	
	2	2	9
	3	2	
	4	6	8
	5	1	
	6	2	3
Total		62	

Example 1
Table 4.1 denotes individual dates of birth of $n = 35$ cases of the birth defects oesophageal atresia and tracheo-oesophageal fistula observed in a hospital in Birmingham, U.K., from 1950 through 1955. Is there any clustering in time?

Example 2
Table 4.2 indicates $n = 62$ cases of trisomy among karyotyped spontaneous abortions of pregnancies by calendar month of the last menstrual period from July 1975 to June 1977 in three New York hospitals. Do the data suggest any temporal cluster of diseases?

4.1 Data

To test for temporal clustering, we need to collect data retrospectively on the *time of occurrence* of each case for a defined geographic region during a specified study period. *Date of onset*, *date of birth*, and *date of death* have been used as the time of occurrence for clustering of diseases. The rationale for using date of onset invokes a short time interval between the inductive event and onset of disease. Needless to say, very great care is required for clustering by date of death for older people because of the long and variable interval between the onset and death. Throughout this chapter, it is assumed that:

1. We have n independent observed cases.
2. If individual time points data are available, a set of observed times are denoted by $\{t_1, t_2, \ldots, t_n\}$ and the distance between the ith and jth time points is defined as $d_{ij} = |t_i - t_j|$.
3. If the study interval is divided into m disjoint subintervals, a set of count data are denoted by $(n_1, \ldots, n_m)$ and $n = n_1 + \cdots + n_m$ and the distance between ith and jth subintervals is defined as $d_{ij} = |i - j|$.

Depending on the study, as in the case of Ederer *et al.*'s (1964) investigation, described later, the study population might be stratified into several m-year periods, say.

4.2 Null Hypothesis vs. Alternative Hypothesis

The null hypothesis of *no clustering in time* and the alternative hypothesis are stated as the following:

$$H_0: \text{ the times of onset (or diagnosis) of the disease under study}$$
$$\text{are randomly distributed across the study interval} \tag{4.1}$$
$$H_1: \text{ not } H_0$$

If the individual time point data $(t_1, \ldots, t_n)$ are available over the specified study period $[0, T]$ where changes in the population at risk are negligible, then the null hypothesis can be restated as follows where $z_i = t_i/T$, $i = 1, \ldots, n$:

$$H_0: (z_1, \ldots, z_n) \text{ are uniformly distributed across the unit interval } (0, 1]$$
$$\tag{4.2}$$

On the other hand, consider a study period divided into several disjoint subintervals where changes in the population at risk are negligible. The number of cases in region i is denoted by the random number N_i with observed number n_i, $i = 1, \ldots, m$. Under the null hypothesis, given n, $(N_1, \ldots, N_m)$ follows a uniform multinomial distribution with parameter $\boldsymbol{p}^t = (p_1, \ldots, p_m)$, $p_i = 1/m, i = 1, \ldots, m$. The multinomial distribution is given by

$$\Pr\{N_1 = n_1, ..., N_m = n_m \mid \boldsymbol{p}' = (p_1, ..., p_m)\} = \frac{n!}{n_1! \cdots n_m!} \prod_{i=1}^{m} p_i^{n_i} \qquad (4.3)$$

Therefore, the hypotheses above can be restated as

$$H_0 : \ (N_1, ..., N_m) \sim \text{Multinomial}(n, \boldsymbol{p}), \ p_i = \frac{1}{m}, \ i = 1, ..., m \qquad (4.4)$$

Regardless of data type, time point data or count data, it depends on the test whether a particular type of alternative hypothesis H_1 is specified or not.

4.3 Historical Overview of Methods

(It should be noted that there are several other proposed methods not mentioned here. Furthermore, readers who are not interested in the history can skip this section.)

Ederer, Myers, and Mantel (1964) developed a test for temporal clustering using a cell-occupancy approach in their paper entitled "Do leukemia cases come in clusters?" They examined 333 cases of leukemia in children under the age of 15 among residents of 169 Connecticut towns during 15 years, 1945–1959. The annual data revealed a clear upward trend over the 15-year period. This trend, however, paralleled the increase in the number of children, hence the leukemia incidence rate has remained stable. In order to adjust for the number of children at risk and also to examine the existence of clusters of childhood leukemia, they divided the data into three groups of five years each, leading to $3 \times 169 = 507$ 5-year town units. They considered that the effect of trend over a 5-year period would tend to be negligible. Then, as an index of clustering, they considered M, the maximum number of cases in a year, and M is summed across all the 5-year periods and across all the towns. The sum is tested by using a single degree of freedom chi-squared test

$$X_1^2 = (\mid \sum M - \sum E(M) \mid -0.5)^2 / \sum \text{Var}(M)$$

In general context, Ederer, Myers, and Mantel divided the time period into m disjoint subintervals. Under the null hypothesis of no clustering, the n cases are randomly distributed among the subintervals (i.e., they are multinomially distributed). The test statistic M is the maximum number of cases occurring in a subinterval; i.e., $M = \max(n_1, ..., n_m)$. In this sense, their test statistic is called a *disjoint statistic*, in comparison with Naus' *scan statistic*. A method for determining the probability of distributing n cases (ball) in m years (cells) is obtained using a cell-occupancy distribution (Feller, 1957). They extend their idea to consider the largest total in two successive years or more. Ederer, Myers, and Mantel (1964) and Mantel, Kryscio, and Myers (1976) provide tables of the exact null distribution of M for selected values of m and n.

Naus (1965) proposed a test for temporal clustering, called a *scan statistic*, that is applicable when individual time point data $(t_1,...,t_n)$ are available. The test statistic S_d, the maximum number of cases observed in any interval of fixed length d, is found by "scanning" all intervals of length d, known as the scanning window of fixed size d, in the time period. In certain cases, this approach is intuitively more appealing than the disjoint interval approach of Ederer, Myers, and Mantel (1964), but more complicated mathematically. However, situations exist for which the disjoint statistic is the more satisfactory choice. A major challenge with the scan statistic has been to find analytical results concerning its statistical significance. Naus (1965) and Huntington and Naus (1975) found this probability. Since the formula is computationally intensive, most literature has been devoted to finding approximations and, when possible, tabulating its tail probabilities (Glaz, Naus, and Wallenstein, 2001). For selected interval lengths, time lengths, and sample sizes, tables of p-values provided by Naus (1966) and Wallenstein (1980) can be used. Knox and Lancashire (1982) found a pragmatic approximation to the p-value, but it was no good. Wallenstein and Neff (1987) proposed a simple but excellent approximation for small p-values such as $p < 0.10$. Let T denote the length of the entire study period and $w = d/T$. Then we have

$$\Pr\{S_d \geq k \mid n, T\} \approx \left(\frac{k}{w} - n - 1\right) b(k \mid n, w) + 2 \sum_{i=k+1}^{n} b(i \mid n, w)$$

where

$$b(i \mid n, w) = \binom{n}{i} w^i (1 - w)^{n-i}$$

Although this formula often gives a poor approximation for larger p-values, it does not matter for a statistical significance at around or less than 0.05. For example, when $n = 62$, $k = 7$, $d = 1$, $T = 24$, in the examples of trisomy data illustrated later, we have $p \approx 1.09 > 1$, indicating that the test result is not significant anyway. Naus compared the power of the scan test with that of the Ederer, Myers, and Mantel (1964) test and concluded that if the scanning interval is small and the data are continuous over the interval, the scan test is the more powerful of the two. Weinstock (1981) considered a generalization of the scan test that adjusts for changes in the population at risk assuming that the population at risk is available at any time. However, it is not easy to obtain the population at risk at any time.

Since unknown d must be chosen without looking at the data, we usually face multiple testing by choosing a number of plausible values. To adjust for multiple testing, Nagarwalla (1996) extended the scan statistic to the one with a variable window, whose size does not need to be chosen *a priori*. Let $(t_1,...,t_n)$ denote a random sample of n points from the density $f(t)$ in an interval $[0, T]$, and consider testing the hypothesis $H_0 : f(x) = 1/T$ against $H_1 : f(x) = 1/T + \delta$ for $a \leq x \leq a+d$. Then, the test is the maximized likelihood ratio test statistic λ that allows for clusters of variable width d

$$\lambda = \sup_{d} \left(\frac{k}{n}\right)^{k} \left(\frac{n-k}{n}\right)^{n-k} \left(\frac{T}{d}\right)^{k} \left(\frac{T}{T-d}\right)^{n-k}$$

where $k = k(a,d)$ is the number of points in the window $(a, a+d]$. Unfortunately, we can always reject H_0 because we can make λ arbitrarily large by choosing d arbitrarily small such that $k(a,d) \geq 1$. In other words, each point can be declared by itself to be a cluster. To avoid this, Nagarwalla (1996) restricted the clusters to have $k \geq n_0$ points for some predetermined n_0. Then, we can find the supremum over all $k \geq n_0$:

$$\lambda = \sup_{d,\, k \geq n_0} \left(\frac{k}{n}\right)^{k} \left(\frac{n-k}{n}\right)^{n-k} \left(\frac{T}{d}\right)^{k} \left(\frac{T}{T-d}\right)^{n-k}$$

Nagarwalla gave a simple algorithm for the implementation of the method, but Monte Carlo hypothesis testing is used to obtain the p-value since it is not possible to obtain the null distribution of λ analytically.

Bailar, Eisenberg, and Mantel (1970) suggested a test for detecting temporal clustering based on the number of pairs of cases in a given area that occur within a specified length of time d of each other. The numbers of close pairs occurring in q areas are summed. The test statistic is assumed to be approximately normally distributed. Larsen, Holmes, and Heath (1973) developed a rank order test for detecting temporal clustering. The time period is divided into disjoint subintervals that are numbered sequentially (i.e., ranked). Their test statistic S is the sum of absolute differences between the rank of the subinterval in which a case occurred and the median subinterval rank. Small values of S indicate unimodal clustering. Generally, the S-statistics for multiple geographic areas are summed. The resulting statistic is asymptotically normal with simple mean and variance. This test is sensitive only to unimodal clustering; it cannot distinguish multiple clustering from randomness.

Tango (1984) developed a test for temporal clustering based on the distribution of counts in m disjoint subintervals where changes in the population at risk are negligible. The test is useful when the data are grouped. The test statistic, known as the clustering index C, is a quadratic form involving the relative frequencies in each interval and a measure of closeness between intervals

$$C = \mathbf{r}' \mathbf{A} \mathbf{r} = \sum_{i=1}^{m} \sum_{j=1}^{m} \frac{n_i n_j}{n^2} a_{ij}, \quad (0 < C \leq 1)$$

where $\mathbf{r}' = (n_1, ..., n_m)/n$ and the entries a_{ij} of the $m \times m$ symmetric matrix $\mathbf{A}$ are arbitrary known measures of closeness between the ith and jth intervals with the property $a_{ii} = 1$ and a_{ij} is a monotonically nonincreasing function of d_{ij}, the time between the ith and jth subintervals. Tango used the following form as a natural choice.

$$a_{ij} = \exp(-d_{ij}) = \exp(-|i-j|)$$

The clustering index obtains a maximum value of 1 when all cases occur in the same interval. Although the statistic is easy to calculate, the originally proposed asymptotic null distribution was rather complex for simple use. Whittemore and Keller (1986) showed that the distribution of Tango's index is asymptotically normal with simple mean and variance. However, later on, Tango (1990) showed that their normal approximation was very poor for moderately large sample sizes and suggested a central Chi-squared distribution with the degrees of freedom adjusted by the skewness as a better approximation. Although not mentioned in his paper, it can provide a statistic to estimate the clustering periods that made large contributions to significant clustering. If the null hypothesis of no clustering is rejected, we can indicate the likely clustering subinterval i with large values of

$$U_i = \frac{1}{C} \sum_{j=1}^{m} \frac{n_i n_j}{n^2} a_{ij}, \quad \left(\sum_{i=1}^{m} U_i = 1 \right)$$

which denote the percentage of the ith subinterval's contribution to the significant clustering. To adjust for changes in the population at risk, we can apply a spatial version of Tango's index (Tango, 2000),

$$C = (r - p)^t A (r - p) = \sum_{i=1}^{m} \sum_{j=1}^{m} \left(\frac{n_i - e_i}{n} \right) \left(\frac{n_j - e_j}{n} \right) a_{ij}$$

where $p = E_{H_0}(r)$ and $e_i = n p_i$, $i = 1, ..., m$.

Kulldorff and Nagarwalla (1995) and Kulldorff (1997) proposed the spatial scan statistic, which is a spatial version of the scan statistic with a variable window size. This spatial scan statistic can be used to detect temporal clustering. Molinari, Bonaldi, and Daures (2001) proposed a test for temporal clustering by applying a piecewise-constant regression model that allows for multiple cluster detection. They used the AIC (Akaike information criterion) and BIC (Bayesian information criterion) to determine the optimal model including the number of clusters. Naus and Wallenstein (2006) proposed the prospective use of the scan statistic for temporal surveillance.

4.4 Selected Methods

In this section, we shall describe the details of selected tests for temporal clustering. The selection criteria are either (1) being *widely known* or (2) being *frequently cited* in the literature.

4.4.1 Ederer-Myers-Mantel's Method for Count Data

Goal: To find the maximum frequency among disjoint subintervals and evaluate the significance. A significantly large value would indicate evidence of temporal clustering of the disease under study in the subinterval with the maximum frequency.
Null hypothesis H_0: (4.4)
Alternative hypothesis H_1: not H_0

Test statistic

$$M = \max(n_1, ..., n_m), \; n = n_1 + \cdots + n_m \tag{4.5}$$

where the study period is divided into m disjoint subintervals and changes in the population at risk are assumed to be negligible over the study period.

Null distribution

The null distribution of M is derived using the cell-occupancy distribution (Feller, 1957). The probability of a set of occupancy numbers, $(n_{(1)} \geq n_{(2)} \geq \cdots \geq n_{(m)})$, arranged in descending order of number of occupying balls, is

$$\Pr\{n_{(1)}, n_{(2)}..., n_{(m)} \mid n\} = \frac{n!}{n_{(1)}! n_{(2)}! \cdots n_{(m)}!} \frac{m!}{k_0! k_1! \cdots k_n!} \left(\frac{1}{m}\right)^n \tag{4.6}$$

where k_j denotes the number of cells containing exactly j balls and we have

$$\sum_{i=1}^{m} n_{(i)} = n, \quad \sum_{j=0}^{n} k_j = m$$

Therefore the null distribution of M is given by

$$\Pr\{M = n_{(1)} \mid n\} = \sum_{(n_{(2)}, ..., n_{(m)})} \Pr\{n_{(1)}, n_{(2)}..., n_{(m)} \mid n\} \tag{4.7}$$

and the p-value is given by

$$p\text{-value} = \Pr\{M \geq n_{(1)} \mid n\} = \sum_{n_{(1)}} \sum_{(n_{(2)}, ..., n_{(m)})} \Pr\{n_{(1)}, n_{(2)}..., n_{(m)} \mid n\} \tag{4.8}$$

For example, let us assume that $m = 5$, $n = 3$, and the maximum frequency is 3. In this case, we can have three distributions: (a) $(3, 0, 0, 0, 0)$, (b) $(2, 1, 0, 0, 0)$, and (c) $(1, 1, 1, 0, 0)$. Their probabilities are as follows:

$$\Pr\{M=3 \mid n=3\} = \Pr\{3,0,0,0,0 \mid n=3\} = \frac{3!}{3!0!0!0!0!} \frac{5!}{1!4!} \left(\frac{1}{5}\right)^3 = 0.04$$

$$\Pr\{M=2 \mid n=3\} = \Pr\{2,1,0,0,0 \mid n=3\} = \frac{3!}{2!1!0!0!0!} \frac{5!}{1!1!3!} \left(\frac{1}{5}\right)^3 = 0.48$$

$$\Pr\{M=1 \mid n=3\} = \Pr\{1,1,1,0,0 \mid n=3\} = \frac{3!}{1!1!1!0!0!} \frac{5!}{3!2!} \left(\frac{1}{5}\right)^3 = 0.48$$

Therefore, the p-value is 0.04. In addition, the expected value and variance of M are calculated as

$$E(M) = 1 \times 0.48 + 2 \times 0.48 + 3 \times 0.04 = 1.56$$
$$\text{Var}(M) = (1-1.56)^2 \times 0.48 + (2-1.56)^2 \times 0.48 + (3-1.56)^2 \times 0.04 = 0.33$$

When M is summed over several regions and time periods, assuming asymptotic normality, the sum can be tested by using a single degree of freedom chi-squared test:

$$X_1^2 = (|\sum M - \sum E(M)| - 0.5)^2 / \sum \text{Var}(M) \tag{4.9}$$

Regarding tables of $E(M)$ and $\text{Var}(M)$ for selected values of m and n, see Ederer, Myers, and Mantel (1964) and Mantel, Kryscio, and Myers (1976). Needless to say, we can apply Monte Carlo hypothesis testing to obtain the null distribution and the Monte Carlo simulated p-value (2.17).

4.4.2 Naus' Scan Statistic for Point Data

Goal: To find the maximum frequency observed in any interval of fixed length and evaluate the significance. A significantly large value would indicate evidence of temporal clustering of the disease under study in the interval of fixed length with the maximum frequency.
Null hypothesis H_0: (4.2)
Alternative hypothesis H_1: not H_0

Test statistic

S_d = the maximum number of cases observed in an interval of fixed length d.

$$\tag{4.10}$$

Null distribution

The null distribution of S_d will be of the form

$$\Pr\{S_d \geq k \mid n, T\} = \Pr\{S_d \geq k \mid (t_1, ..., t_n) \sim \text{Uniform}(0, T)\} \tag{4.11}$$

A simple and easy-to-compute good approximation was proposed by Wallenstein and Neff (1987),

$$\Pr\{S_d \geq k \mid n, T\} \approx \left(\frac{k}{w} - n - 1\right) b(k \mid n, w) + 2 \sum_{i=k+1}^{n} b(i \mid n, w) \quad (4.12)$$

where $w = d/T$ and

$$b(i \mid n, w) = \binom{n}{i} w^i (1 - w)^{n-i} \quad (4.13)$$

Needless to say, we can apply Monte Carlo hypothesis testing to obtain the null distribution and the Monte Carlo simulated p-value (2.17).

4.4.3 Nagarwalla's Scan Statistic for Point Data

Goal: To find the most likely hot-spot cluster in the study period and evaluate the significance. Detection of a significant hot-spot cluster would indicate evidence of the existence of a temporal cluster of disease under study.

Null hypothesis and alternative hypothesis
Let $(z_1, ..., z_n)$, $z_i = 1/T$, denote a random sample of n points from the density $f(t)$, which expresses a "hot-spot" cluster on a line:

$$f(t) = \begin{cases} \frac{1}{T} + \delta & \text{for } a \leq t \leq a+d \\ \frac{1}{T} - \delta \frac{d}{T-d} & \text{for } 0 \leq t < a \text{ or } a+d < t \leq 1. \end{cases} \quad (4.14)$$

Then the null hypothesis and the alternative hypothesis are reexpressed by

$$H_0: \ \delta = 0, \ H_1: \delta > 0 \quad (4.15)$$

Test statistic

Under the formulation above, Nagarwalla's scan statistic is a likelihood ratio test statistic

$$\lambda = \sup_{d, \ k \geq n_0} \left(\frac{k}{n}\right)^k \left(\frac{n-k}{n}\right)^{n-k} \left(\frac{T}{d}\right)^k \left(\frac{T}{T-d}\right)^{n-k} \quad (4.16)$$

where $k = k(a, d)$ is the number of points in the window $(a, \ a+d]$ and n_0 is a predetermined lowest number of cases for clusters. Nagarwalla (1996) gave the following simple algorithm for the implementation of the method:

For each $k = n_0, ..., n-2$
   For each $i = 1, ..., n-k+1$
      Find: $(x_{i+k-1} - x_i)$
    Let $d_{\min}[k] = \min_i(x_{i+k-1} - x_i)$
     $i_{\min}[k] = \{i : d_{\min}[k] = (x_{i+k-1} - x_i)\}$
    Find

$$\lambda[k] = \left(\frac{k}{n}\right)^k \left(\frac{n-k}{n}\right)^{n-k} \left(\frac{T}{d}\right)^k \left(\frac{T}{T-d}\right)^{n-k}$$

Let $\lambda^* = \max_k \lambda[k]$, and let k^* and i^* be the values
for which the maximum is achieved.

Null distribution

Monte Carlo hypothesis testing is required to obtain the null distribution of *lambda* and the Monte Carlo simulated *p*-value (2.17).

4.4.4 Kulldorff's Scan Statistic for Count Data

This test is a temporal version of the spatial scan statistic developed by Kulldorff and Nagarwalla (1995) and Kulldorff (1997). For details, see Chapter 5.

Goal: To detect the most likely hot-spot cluster within the study interval divided into several disjoint subintervals and evaluate the significance. The finding that the most likely cluster is significant would suggest evidence for the existence of a temporal cluster within the study area. This method can adjust for the heterogeneity of population at risk over the study interval.

Null hypothesis and alternative hypothesis
Let us assume that

$$(N_1, ..., N_m) \sim \text{Multinomial}(n, \boldsymbol{p}), \ \boldsymbol{p}^t = (p_1, ..., p_m) \tag{4.17}$$

where

$$p_i = \frac{\xi_i}{\sum_{j=1}^m \xi_j}, \ i = 1, ..., m \tag{4.18}$$

and ξ_i denotes the population at risk in subinterval i, and the expected number of cases in subinterval i is $e_i = np_i$. Then the null hypothesis and the alternative hypothesis are reexpressed by

$$H_0: \ E(N(J)) = e(J), \quad \text{for all } J$$
$$H_1: \ E(N(J)) > e(J), \quad \text{for some } J$$

where $J = [s, s+k-1]$, an interval of length k, and $N(J)$ and $e(J) = \sum_{i \in J} n p_i$ denote the random number of cases and the null expected number of cases within the specified interval J, respectively. Under the alternative hypothesis, there is an elevated risk within some interval J compared with outside it.

Test statistic

The test statistic is the likelihood ratio maximized for J similar to Nagarwalla's scan statistic for continuous data

$$\lambda = \sup_{J} \left(\frac{n(J)}{e(J)} \right)^{n(J)} \left(\frac{n-n(J)}{n-e(J)} \right)^{n-n(J)} I\left(\frac{n(J)}{e(J)} > \frac{n-n(J)}{n-e(J)} \right) \qquad (4.19)$$

where $n(J)$ and $e(J)$ denote the observed number and the null expected number of cases within the interval J and $I()$ is the indicator function. The interval J^* that attains the maximum likelihood is defined as the *most likely cluster* (MLC).

Null distribution

Monte Carlo hypothesis testing is required to obtain the null distribution of λ and the Monte Carlo simulated p-value (2.17). To apply this test, version 8 of a free software package called SaTScan developed by Kulldorff and Information Management Services (2009) can be used.

4.4.5 Tango's Index for Count Data

Goal: To calculate the clustering index with a measure of closeness between subintervals and evaluate the significance. A significantly large value would indicate evidence of temporal clustering of the disease under study.
Null hypothesis H_0: (4.4)
Alternative hypothesis H_1: not H_0

Test statistic

The test statistic is

$$C = r^t A r = \sum_{i=1}^{m} \sum_{j=1}^{m} \frac{n_i n_j}{n^2} a_{ij} \qquad (4.20)$$

where $r^t = (n_1, ..., n_m)/n$ and a_{ij} is a *measure of closeness* between the ith and jth subintervals:

$$a_{ij} = \exp(-|i-j|) \qquad (4.21)$$

Null distribution

The p-value can be obtained using the good approximation

$$\Pr\{C > c \mid H_0\} \approx \Pr\left\{\chi_v^2 > v + \sqrt{2v}\left(\frac{c - E(C)}{\sqrt{\text{Var}(C)}}\right)\right\} \qquad (4.22)$$

where

$$E(C) = m^{-2}\{1'A1 + n^{-1}\text{tr}[AV]\}$$
$$\text{Var}(C) = m^{-4}n^{-1}\{41'AVA1 + 2n^{-2}\text{tr}[(AV)^2]\}$$
$$v = 8/(\sqrt{\beta_1(C)})^2$$
$$\sqrt{\beta_1(C)} = \frac{8\{31'(AV)^2A1 + n^{-1}\text{tr}[(AV)^3]\}}{\sqrt{n}\{41'AVA1 + 2n^{-1}\text{tr}[(AV)^2]\}^{3/2}}$$
$$1 = (1, ..., 1)' \ (\text{length } m)$$
$$V = \text{diag}(m1) - 11'$$

where $\text{diag}(x)$ is the $m \times m$ diagonal matrix with the vector x. The approximation above is fairly accurate even for small n. The Monte Carlo simulated p-value (2.17) can be obtained by applying Monte Carlo hypothesis testing to the standardized test statistic

$$Z = \frac{C - E(C)}{\sqrt{\text{Var}(C)}}$$

Identifying likely clusters

If the null hypothesis of no clustering is rejected, we can indicate the likely clustering subinterval i with large values of

$$U_i = \frac{1}{C}\sum_{j=1}^{m}\frac{n_i n_j}{n^2}a_{ij}, \qquad \left(\sum_{i=1}^{m}U_i = 1\right) \qquad (4.23)$$

which denote the percentage of the ith subinterval's contribution to the significant clustering.

Heterogeneous population at risk

If changes in the population at risk are not negligible, then calculate the null probability p_i defined in (4.18) and use the test statistic

$$C_S = (r - p)'A(r - p) = \sum_{i=1}^{m}\sum_{j=1}^{m}\left(\frac{n_i - e_i}{n}\right)\left(\frac{n_j - e_j}{n}\right)a_{ij} \qquad (4.24)$$

where $p = E_{H_0}(r)$ and $e_i = np_i$, $i = 1,...,m$. We shall omit further explanations here. For details, see Chapter 5.

4.5 Illustration with Real Data

Two published data sets were used to illustrate some of the methods selected in the previous section. In these examples, it is assumed that changes in the population at risk are negligible during the study period.

4.5.1 Congenital Oesophageal Atresia Data

The first data set we use consists of individual dates of birth of $n = 35$ cases of the birth defects oesophageal atresia and tracheo-oesophageal fistula observed in a hospital in Birmingham, U.K., between 1950 and 1955 ($T = 2191$). It was first published by Knox (1959) and subsequently analyzed by Weinstock (1981) using a scan statistic with a fixed window and by Nagarwalla (1996) using a scan statistic with a variable window. The data are shown in Table 4.1, and the second column is the number of days past 1 January 1950 on which each case was observed. The third, fourth, and fifth columns of the table denote the frequency of cases per 100 days, 200 days, and 365 days (one year), respectively. It seems probable that there occur three close subintervals [1200, 1299], [1300, 1399], [1400, 1499] and another less striking concentration in the last three subintervals [1900, 1999], [2000, 2099], [2100, 2190]. We shall show the results of applying the scan statistic with a window of fixed length, the scan statistic with a window of variable length, and the clustering index.

Naus' scan statistic for point data

1. Fixed length $d = 100$:

   $S_d = 7$ for the cluster of seven cases from day 1233 (17 May 1953) to day 1305 (28 July 1953). $w = 7/2191 = 0.0456$. Using Wallenstein and Neff's approximation (4.12), we obtain $p \approx 0.088$. Output from the R program is shown below.

R program of Wallenstein and Neff's approximation

```
> n < - 35; k < - 7; d < - 100; t < - 2191
> w < - d/t
> w
[1] 0.04564126
> (k/w - n - 1) * dbinom(k, n, w) + 2 * (1 - pbinom(k, n, w))
[1] 0.08832566
```

---

2. Fixed window $d = 200$

   $S_d = 10$ for the cluster of ten cases from day 1233 (17 May 1953) to day 1390 (21 October 1953). Using the approximation (4.12), we obtain $p \approx 0.0499$.

3. Fixed window $d = 300$

   $S_d = 15$ for the cluster of 15 cases from day 1233 (17 May 1953) to day 1491 (30 January 1954). Using the approximation (4.12), we obtain $p \approx 0.0014$.

4. Fixed window $d = 365$

   Weinstock (1981) applied the Naus scan statistic with $d = 365$ to these data. $S_d = 16$ for the cluster of 16 cases from day 1233 (17 May 1953) to day 1583 (2 May 1954). Using the approximation (4.12), we obtain $p \approx 0.0027$. Results of four different scan statistics with fixed windows $d = 100$, 200, 300, and 365 suggest the optimal window size could be between 200 and 365.

Nagarwalla's scan statistic for point data

Nagarwalla (1996) set $n_0 = 5$ and computed the maximum likelihood ratio (4.16). $\lambda^* = 43968$ and the most likely cluster is the set of 15 cases from day 1233 (17 May 1953) to day 1491 (30 January 1954), which is the same as that of the scan statistic with fixed window $d = 300$. The optimal and minimum window is $1491 - 1233 + 1 = 259$. Using Monte Carlo testing with $N_{rep} = 9999$ repetitions, the observed rank of λ^* from Nagarwalla's computation is 58, i.e., $p = 0.0058$. An output from the R function **Nagarwalla.test** (Appendix) for Nagarwalla's scan statistic with a Monte Carlo simulated p-value with 9999 repetitions is shown below, which tells us that the observed test statistic is the log-likelihood ratio $\log \lambda = 10.69122 = $**out\$Nagarwalla.T** $(\exp(10.69122) = 43,968)$ with simulated $p = 0.0073$ (see Figure 4.1). The most likely cluster is the set of $15 = $**out\$kstar** cases from the day $1233 = $**out\$MLCfrom** to the day $1491 = $**out\$MLCto**.

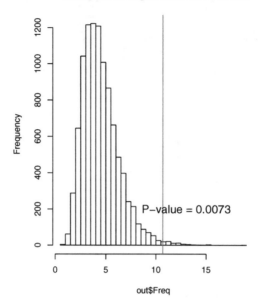

Fig. 4.1 Histogram of the simulated Nagarwalla scan statistic T based on Monte Carlo hypothesis testing with $N_{rep} = 9999$ repetitions and the location of the observed Nagarwalla scan statistic.

Output from the R function Nagarwalla.test

```
> n0< − 5; tt< − 2191; Nrep< − 9999
> out< − Nagarwalla.test(yday,tt,n0,Nrep)
> out$Nagarwalla.T:
[1] 10.69122
> out$Simulated.p.value:
[1] 0.0073
> out$kstar:
[1] 15
> out$MLCfrom:
[1] 1233
> out$MLCto:
[1] 1491
```

Output from the R function TangoT.index

> Nrep< −9999
> f100< −c(0,1,0,1,2,0,0,0,0,1,1,1,6,4,5,1,1,2,0,2,4,3)
> TangoT.index(Nrep, f100)
out$Stnd.C:
[1] 5.01574
out$C.p.value:
[1] 0.0002713008 ········· approximation (4.22)
out$MC.p.value:
[1] 0.0004
out$C.u:
[1,] 0.000000000 ········· interval 0–99
[2,] 0.006020562
[3,] 0.000000000
[4,] 0.009140527
[5,] 0.023687112
[6,] 0.000000000
[7,] 0.000000000
[8,] 0.000000000
[9,] 0.000000000
[10,] 0.009401614
[11,] 0.013916686 ········ interval 1000–1099
[12,] 0.022094544
[13,] 0.256905956
[14,] 0.165319105
[15,] 0.194603871
[16,] 0.021521108
[17,] 0.016043857
[18,] 0.033079682
[19,] 0.000000000
[20,] 0.041573321
[21,] 0.116600904 ········ interval 2000–2099
[22,] 0.070091150

Tango's index for count data

1. Count data per 100 days

   Output from the R function **TangoT.index** (Appendix) for Tango's index for temporal clustering assuming a homogeneous population at risk is shown above. The observed standardized clustering index is **Stnd.C** = 5.015, and using the approximation (4.22), we obtain **C.p.value** ≈ 0.00027. The Monte Carlo sim-

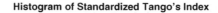

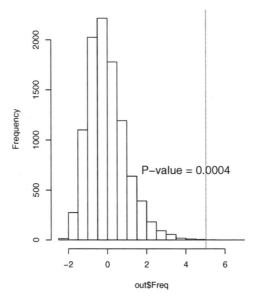

Fig. 4.2 Histogram of the simulated standardized Tango index C based on Monte Carlo hypothesis testing with $N_{rep} = 9999$ repetitions and the location of the observed value of Tango's index.

ulated p-value with $N_{rep} = 9999$ is **MC.p.value**= 0.0004 (see Figure 4.2). By examining the percentage contribution of U_i to C (**C.u**), we can see that three successive subintervals, 13 : $[1200, 1299]$, 14 : $[1300, 1399]$, 15 : $[1400, 1499]$ (15 cases from day 1233 to day 1491), have quite large values compared with those of other subintervals, and their contribution is 61.7%, indicating a strong clustering period in these three successive subintervals. Furthermore, we can observe another clustering period in two successive subintervals, 21 : $[2000, 2099]$, 22 : $[2100, 2199]$ (seven cases from day 2049 to the last day, 2174), which contributed about 18.7%.

2. Count data per 200 days

   The observed standardized clustering index is $C = 5.222$, the approximated p-value (4.22) is $p \approx 0.00046$, and the simulated p-value is 0.0005. By examining the percentage contribution of U_i to C, we can see a cluster in the two successive subintervals $[1200, 1399], [1400, 1599]$ (16 cases from day 1233 to day 1583) that has a 61.8% contribution. Furthermore, we can observe another clustering period in the last subinterval $[2000, 2199]$ (seven cases from day 2049 to the last day 2174), which contributed about 18.0%.

3. Count data per one year (365 days)

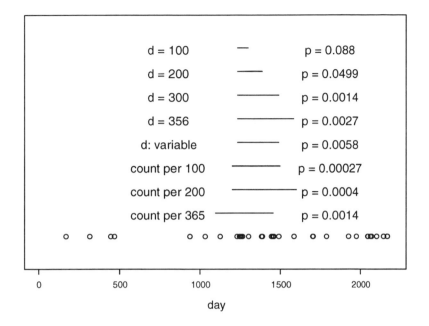

Fig. 4.3 Intervals of significant clustering detected or considered to have a large contribution to significant clustering by each of eight methods and the resultant *p*-values.

The observed standardized clustering index is $C = 4.745$, and using the approximation (4.22), we obtain $p \approx 0.0014$. The simulated *p*-value is 0.0007. By examining the percentage contribution of U_i to C, we can see a cluster in the subinterval $[1095, 1459]$ (14 cases from day 1128 to day 1458) that has about a 51.3% contribution. Furthermore, we can observe another clustering period in the last subinterval $[1825, 2190]$ (nine cases from day 1924 to the last day, 2174), which contributed about 23.6%.

Summary

Figure 4.3 shows eight time intervals of the significant clusters detected by each of eight different methods. Needless to say, it should be noted that the last three intervals were not those *detected* by Tango's index. This figure shows that most of the intervals, except for those of the two cases $d = 100$ and $d = 200$ of Naus' scan statistic, commonly include the interval $[1233, 1491]$ detected by Nagarwalla's scan statistic and Naus' scan statistic with $d = 300$. Therefore, it appears most likely that the clustering has occurred in this interval. This figure also clearly shows that Naus' scan statistic with a small d cannot detect a larger cluster. Needless to say, when we do not have any information on the choice of d, we usually face multiple testing by repeating the procedure, choosing a number of plausible values as in the examples above. In this sense, Nagarwalla's scan statistic with a window of variable length can be recommended. However, as the example above shows, all the p-values of Tango's index are smaller than that of Nagarwalla's scan statistic. Tango's index is usually more powerful than Nagarwalla's scan statistic from my experience (data not shown here) due to the property that the former utilizes the frequency data adjacent to the interval with the maximum frequency by using a measure of closeness defined in (4.21), while the latter uses the maximum frequency data only. Needless to say, the result of Tango's index will depend on the way of grouping continuous data, as in the case of count data per 365 days.

4.5.2 Trisomy Data

The second data set consists of $n = 62$ cases of trisomy among karyotyped spontaneous abortions of pregnancies, by calendar month of the last menstrual period from July 1975 to June 1977, in three New York hospitals. The data are shown in Table 4.2, where the trisomy data are tabulated in two ways: (1) monthly over 24 months and (2) bimonthly over 24 months. Visual inspection of the data suggests that a cluster seems to occur during the period November 1976 to January 1977.

It was first analyzed by Wallenstein (1980) and subsequently analyzed by Tango (1984, 1990). Wallenstein (1980) applied Naus' scan statistic to individual trisomy data (not shown in his paper). In his illustration, he set $d = 60$ days and found $S_d = 14$, $p = 0.038$ based on his unpublished extensive table. Linear interpolation based on his Table 1 yields $p = 0.040$. Using the approximation (4.12), we obtain $p = 0.037$. In the tabulated data, the maximum number of trisomies in two consecutive months was also 14. In general, inspection of *all* 60-day intervals may yield a higher value than the maximum number from two consecutive months.

As the Edere-Myers-Mantel method is computationally intensive and its power is usually less than Tango's index and Kulldorff's scan statistic, we shall illustrate here Tango's index and Kulldorff's scan statistic with the tabulated trisomy data.

Tango's index

Based on the approximation (4.22), Tango (1984, 1990) examined the following three cases. All the results are significant at the 5% level: (a) for monthly data over 24 months, $C = 0.1139$, $p \approx 0.023$ (simulated p-value 0.0219 with $N_{rep} = 9999$); (b) for bimonthly data over 24 months, $C = 0.1975$, $p \approx 0.035$ (simulated p-value 0.0304); and (c) for monthly data over the last 12 months, $C = 0.2354$, $p \approx 0.0046$ (simulated p-value 0.0035). In the case of (a), using U_i, we can find a likely cluster in the period from November 1976 to January 1977, which has 18 cases and a 45.5% contribution.

Kulldorff's scan statistic (using SaTScan)

We show the results for monthly count data over 24 months using SaTScan. A part of
the output of SaTScan is shown below. The most likely cluster is the set of 28 cases
from November 1976 to April 1977. Using Monte Carlo testing with 999 replicates,
the observed rank of the log-likelihood ratio statistic is 22; i.e., $p = 0.022$.

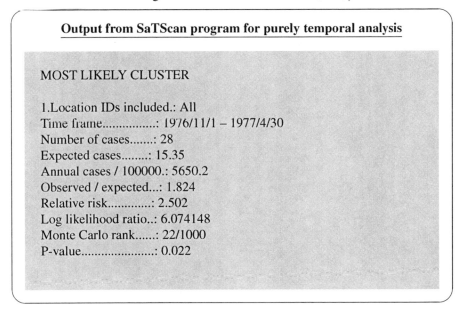

Output from SaTScan program for purely temporal analysis

MOST LIKELY CLUSTER

1.Location IDs included.: All
Time frame...............: 1976/11/1 − 1977/4/30
Number of cases.......: 28
Expected cases........: 15.35
Annual cases / 100000.: 5650.2
Observed / expected...: 1.824
Relative risk.............: 2.502
Log likelihood ratio..: 6.074148
Monte Carlo rank......: 22/1000
P-value.....................: 0.022

4.6 Discussion

The Ederer-Myers-Mantel method for count data has been widely used in epidemiological studies, probably because its simple single degree of freedom chi-squared
test statistic (4.9) can easily be applied to stratified data given tables for the exact distribution of M. However, its power is usually low because their test statistic
is the maximum frequency among the predefined subintervals. Therefore, a more
powerful test statistic could be

$$X^2 = \left(\sum C - \sum E(C)\right)^2 / \sum \text{Var}(C) \tag{4.25}$$

where C is Tango's index C. However, as I am not sure whether asymptotic normality
can be assumed for the sum $\sum C$, Monte Carlo hypothesis testing will be required to
obtain the null distribution.

Naus' scan statistic for point data is mathematically interesting and thus has attracted much interest in the literature. However, its practical application to epidemiological studies strongly faces multiple testing problems of repeating the analysis by

choosing a number of plausible values of temporal window d. So, to avoid multiplicity of testing, Nagarwalla's scan statistic with a variable window is recommended. As the corresponding method for count data, Kulldorff's scan statistic can be used. These two scan statistics try to find the most likely hot-spot cluster. To find the other type of clustering, a *clinal cluster*, which is observed more often than a hot-spot cluster, Tango's index can be a good alternative for count data.

Chapter 5
General Tests for Spatial Clustering: Regional Count Data

We shall consider here the problem of detecting disease clustering in space based on regional count data, which is illustrated by the following two examples.

Example 1

Figure 5.1 shows a choropleth map of the SMR (standardized mortality ratio) of gallbladder cancer (male) in three adjacent prefectures, Niigata, Fukushima, and

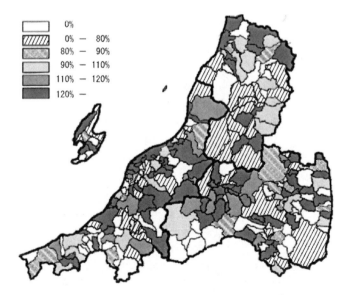

Fig. 5.1 Choropleth map of standardized mortality ratios (SMR) of gallbladder cancer (male) in three adjacent prefectures, Niigata, Fukushima, and Yamagata, consisting of 246 villages, towns, and cities in Japan for the years 1996–2000, based on the age-specific mortality rates from the three prefectures combined.

T. Tango, *Statistical Methods for Disease Clustering*,
Statistics for Biology and Health, DOI 10.1007/978-1-4419-1572-6_5,
© Springer Science+Business Media, LLC 2010

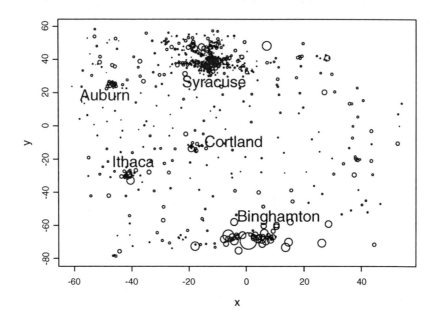

Fig. 5.2 Geographical locations of major cities and 592 leukemia cases in the eight-county region. Circles are drawn only for the census tracts whose observed/expected ratio is statistically significantly larger than 1.0 at $\alpha = 0.05$. The radius is set inversely proportional to the tail probability.

Yamagata, consisting of 246 villages, towns, and cities, Japan for the years 1996–2000, based on the age-specific mortality rates from the three prefectures combined. This is the same map as in Figure 3.4. Does this figure suggest any cluster(s) of gallbladder cancer?

Example 2

Figure 5.2 shows geographical locations of major cities and 592 incident leukemia cases from 1978 to 1982 for each of 790 census tracts among 1,057,673 people at risk in an eight-county region of upstate New York (Waller *et al.*, 1992,1994). Circles are drawn only for the census tracts whose O/E (observed/expected) ratio is statistically significantly larger than 1.0 at $\alpha = 0.05$. The area is set inversely proportional to the tail probability. Are there clusters of leukemia around five major cities?

5.1 Data

To test for spatial clustering using regional count data, we need to collect data on the location of each case for a defined geographic area during a specified study period. Throughout this chapter, it is assumed that:

1. The total observed number of cases is n.
2. The study area is divided into m geographic regions (e.g., census tracts, counties, or states), where:

   a. The number of cases of the disease under study in region i is denoted by n_i with $n = n_1 + \cdots + n_m$.
   b. The population size of region i is denoted by ξ_i.
   c. The centroid of region i is denoted by (x_i, y_i).
   d. The distance between the ith and jth regions is defined as

$$d_{ij} = \sqrt{(x_i - x_j)^2 + (y_i - y_j)^2}$$

5.2 Null Hypothesis vs. Alternative Hypothesis

The null hypothesis of *no clustering in space* and the alternative hypothesis can be simply stated as follows:

H_0 : the locations of onset (or diagnosis or death) of the disease under study

are randomly distributed across the study region (5.1)

H_1 : not H_0

Statistically speaking, we can restate this as follows. Consider a study area divided into m regions. The number of cases in region i is denoted by the random number N_i with observed number n_i, $i = 1, ..., m$. Then, the null hypothesis of no clustering for a rare disease can be expressed as

H_0 : the N_i are independent Poisson variables, with the mean proportional

to the population size ξ_i in region i (5.2)

In other words,

$$H_0 : \ N_i \sim \text{Poisson}(\lambda \xi_i), \ N_i \text{ and } N_j \text{ are independent} \tag{5.3}$$

where λ represents the baseline disease rate, which is *unknown* in general. However, under H_0, the total number $N = N_1 + \cdots + N_m$ of cases is a sufficient statistic for the unknown parameter λ. Therefore a test statistic whose distribution is independent of the unknown parameter λ is obtained by conditioning the total number of cases $N = n$. Given n, the null hypothesis can be

$$H_0 : \ (N_1, ..., N_m) \sim \text{Multinomial}(n, \boldsymbol{p}) \tag{5.4}$$

where

$$\boldsymbol{p}^t = (p_1, ..., p_m), \ p_i = \frac{\xi_i}{\sum_{j=1}^m \xi_j} \tag{5.5}$$

One procedure to adjust for the effect of confounding factors such as sex and age is to partition the population into K categories and assume that diseases occur in each stratum as an independent Poisson process. Then the numbers N_{ik} in the kth category of the confounding factor of the ith region are mutually independent Poisson variables and the null hypothesis (5.3) becomes

$$H_0 : \ N_{ik} \sim \text{Poisson}(\lambda_k \xi_{ik}), \ (i = 1, ..., m, k = 1, ..., K) \tag{5.6}$$

where ξ_{ik} denotes the population size for the kth category of the confounding factor in the ith region. In a similar way, given the marginal number of cases for each category $(n_{+1}, n_{+2}, ..., n_{+K})$, the vector of observed frequencies $(n_{1k}, n_{2k}, ..., n_{mk})$ can be a random sample of size $n_{+k} = n_{1k} + n_{2k} + \cdots + n_{mk}$ from a multinomial distribution with parameter vector $\boldsymbol{p}_k$:

$$\boldsymbol{p}_k^t = (p_{1k}, ..., p_{mk}), \ p_{ik} = \frac{\xi_{ik}}{\sum_{j=1}^m \xi_{jk}} \tag{5.7}$$

Therefore, the parameters p_i of the multinomial distribution under the null hypothesis (5.4) are given by

$$p_i = \sum_{k=1}^K \frac{n_{+k}}{n} p_{ik} = \frac{1}{n} \left(\sum_{k=1}^K \xi_{ik} \frac{\sum_{j=1}^m n_{jk}}{\sum_{j=1}^m \xi_{jk}} \right) \tag{5.8}$$

and the *conditional* null expected number of cases in region i is $e_i = np_i$. In this conditional case, we have

$$n = \sum_{i=1}^m n_i = \sum_i^m e_i \tag{5.9}$$

The other procedure to adjust for the effect of the confounding factor will be to use the standard regression models. Let e_i^R denote the conditional covariate-adjusted null expected number of cases e_{it}^R based on some regression model. Then, we can set

$$p_i = \frac{e_{it}^R}{\sum_{i=1}^m e_i^R} \tag{5.10}$$

so that $\sum_{i=1}^m e_i = \sum_{i=1}^m np_i = n$.

5.3 Historical Overview of Methods

(It should be noted that there are several other proposed methods not mentioned here. Furthermore, readers who are not interested in the history can skip this section.)

Adjacency methods

In the 1950s, two famous global indices of *spatial autocorrelation* came into existence in the literature that assess whether rates for adjacent areas are more similar (i.e., the pattern is clustered) than would be expected if they were randomly distributed among the geographic areas. The most widely used index is Moran's I (Moran, 1950), in which the similarity between regions is defined as the product of the respective *deviations*

$$I = \frac{\sum_{i=1}^{m} \sum_{j=1}^{m} w_{ij}(r_i - \bar{r})(r_j - \bar{r})}{w_{..} \sum_{i=1}^{m} (r_i - \bar{r})^2 / m}$$

where r_i denotes the rate in region i and w_{ij} denotes a measure of adjacency between region i and region j and is defined as

$$w_{ij} = \begin{cases} 1, & \text{region } i \text{ and region } j \text{ are adjacent, } (i \neq j) \\ 0, & \text{otherwise} \end{cases}$$

When neighboring regions tend to have similar rates, I will be positive. When neighboring regions tend to have different rates, I will be negative.

Geary (1954) developed another test of spatial clustering, called *Geary's contiguity ratio c*, which is the ratio of the sum of mean squared differences between rates for pairs of adjacent areas to the weighted sum of mean squared differences between rates for all pairs of areas,

$$c = \frac{m-1}{2m} \frac{\sum_{i=1}^{m} \sum_{j=1}^{m} w_{ij}(r_i - r_j)^2}{w_{..} \sum_{i=1}^{m} (r_i - \bar{r})^2 / m}$$

If the rates are geographically distributed at random, the contiguity ratio is close to one. Low values less than one indicate positive autocorrelation. Geary derived an expression for the approximate variance of the ratio. If the number of areas is not too small, the ratio is asymptotically normally distributed.

Ohno, Aoki, and Aoki (1979) and Ohno and Aoki (1981) developed a simple test for spatial clustering that uses categorized rates that are normally displayed by different colors in disease maps. Their test assesses whether the rates in adjacent areas are more similar than would be expected under the null hypothesis of no clustering. For this test, the rate for each area is classified into one of K categories, and each pair of adjacent areas is identified. The test statistic is the number of adjacent concordant pairs A_k; i.e., the number of pairs of areas that are adjacent and have rates in the same kth category,

$$A_k = \frac{1}{2} \sum_{i=1}^{m} \sum_{j=1}^{m} w_{ij} \delta_{ij(k)}$$

where

$$\delta_{ij(k)} = \begin{cases} 1, \text{ region } i \text{ and region } j \text{ have the same } k\text{th color, } (i \neq j) \\ 0, \text{ otherwise} \end{cases}$$

Then, an overall test statistic is defined by the chi-squared test

$$\chi^2 = \sum_{k=1}^{K} \frac{(A_k - E_k)^2}{E_k}, \quad E_k = \frac{w_{..} m_k (m_k - 1)}{2m(m-1)}$$

where m_k denotes the number of regions in category k. However, there is no statistical guarantee that we can apply the usual asymptotic chi-squared distribution with $K - 1$ degrees of freedom. So, Monte Carlo testing is required for this test.

Grimson, Wang, and Johnson (1981) proposed a test of spatial clustering for use in detecting clusters of geographic areas designated as high risk. The null hypothesis is that high-risk areas are randomly distributed within a larger area and do not cluster. Given m_1 high-risk areas, the test statistic is the number of pairs of high-risk areas that are adjacent to each other. This statistic is equivalent to the category-specific statistic from Ohno, Aoki, and Aoki (1979). Grimson, Wang, and Johnson (1981) recommended using a simple Monte Carlo hypothesis testing to obtain a p-value for the test statistic.

It should be noted, however, that, although these above-stated tests based on adjacencies are easy to use, they do not properly take into account differences in sampling variability of rates due to population heterogeneity. So, they are not recommended in the sense that they may produce spurious results in practice. Oden (1995), Waldhor (1996), and Assuncao and Reis (1999) independently consider modification of Moran's I for incidence proportions and provide derivations of the associated null distribution in the presence of heterogeneous regional population sizes. On the other hand, Walter (1992a, 1992b) suggested adjusting Moran's I for regional counts by comparing the observed count in region i with its expected number under the null hypothesis of no clustering,

$$I_W = \sum_{i=1}^{m} \sum_{j=1}^{m} w_{ij} \frac{n_i - e_i}{\sqrt{e_i}} \frac{n_j - e_j}{\sqrt{e_j}}$$

Distance methods

Whittemore *et al.* (1987) developed a test for spatial clustering across geographic areas that adjusts for different distributions of population subgroups across the study area. The test statistic is the mean distance between all pairs of cases,

$$W = r' D r$$

where $r' = (n_1, \ldots, n_m)/n$ denotes a vector of the observed relative frequencies and W is identical in form to Tango's index in time C (4.20), and thus their test was expressed as a generalization of Tango's index. However, there is an important difference that $D = (d_{ij})$ is used as a measure of distance in Whittemore *et al.*'s test, while $A = (-\exp(d_{ij}))$ was used as a measure of closeness in Tango's index. They proved the asymptotic distribution of this index to be normal and insisted that the clustering index C (4.20) also has an asymptotic normal distribution. However, it does depend largely on the element of A or D used. When the distance measure D is used, convergence to normality is very fast. On the contrary, when the closeness measure A is used, the speed is shown to be too slow and thus normality is not valid even for fairly large sample sizes such as $n = 1000$ (Tango, 1990). Furthermore, more substantially, it has been shown that (1) the quadratic form in $(r - p)$ should be used to properly adjust for heterogeneous populations and (2) due to the selection of D instead of A, the power of W often falls lower than the nominal α level, depending on the clustering model (Tango, 1995, 1999). To see its inappropriateness, the example used in Tango (1995) is shown here. Let us consider the study area comprising three regions with $d_{12} = d_{13} = d_{23}$ and $p = E_{H_0}(r) = (0.2, 0.3, 0.5)^t$. Then consider the two observed cases: (i) $r = (0.2, 0.3, 0.5)^t$ and (ii) $r = (0.5, 0.3, 0.2)^t$. In case (i), we have $r = p$ and we can see there is no clustering. In case (ii), on the other hand, we can observe that the first region has an increased rate compared with other regions. However, the test statistic W produces the same value in both cases. Therefore, Whittemore *et al.*'s test cannot be recommended for practical use.

Tango (1995) proposed a test for spatial clustering with the same purpose as Whittemore *et al.*'s test:

$$C = (r - p)^t A (r - p)$$
$$= \sum_{i=1}^{m} \sum_{j=1}^{m} \left(\frac{n_i - e_i}{n} \right) \left(\frac{n_j - e_j}{n} \right) a_{ij}$$

This test is also called Tango's excess events test (EET) in the literature (e.g., Kulldorff, Tango, and Park, 2003; Song and Kulldorff, 2003, 2005; Pfeiffer *et al.*, 2008). This is an extension of Tango's index for temporal clustering to spatial clustering in that it allows for heterogeneous population size and confounding factors based on indirect standardization. As a measure of closeness $A = (a_{ij})$ between the regions i and j, Tango (1995, 2000) recommended the double exponential clinal type

$$a_{ij} = \exp \left\{ -4 \left(\frac{d_{ij}}{\lambda} \right)^2 \right\}$$

where λ is a measure of *cluster size* and is essentially equal to the maximum distance between cases such that any pair of cases far apart beyond the distance λ cannot be considered a cluster. Large λ will give a test sensitive to a large cluster and small λ a test sensitive to a small cluster. In practical applications, it is rare that we can predict the cluster size before examining the data. Therefore, we usually repeat the procedure using different parameter settings and, consequently, face multiple testing problems. To take this problem into account, Tango (2000) proposed, as an extended test statistic, *the minimum of the profile p-value of C for* λ where λ varies continuously from a small value near zero upward until λ reaches about one-fourth the maximum distance d_{ij} in the study area. The proposed test statistic $P_{\min}$ is defined as

$$P_{\min} = \min_{\lambda} \Pr\{C > c \mid H_0, \lambda\} = \Pr\{C > c \mid H_0, \lambda = \lambda^*\}$$

where λ^* attains the minimum *p*-values of C. The practical implementation of this procedure is to use "line search" by discretizing λ. The null distribution of $P_{\min}$ can be obtained by Monte Carlo hypothesis testing. This approach is also called Tango's MEET (maximized excess events test) in the literature and is quite similar to Baker's (1996) Max test for space-time interaction.

Given λ and under the null hypothesis H_0, the test statistic C can be asymptotically approximated by a chi-squared distribution in the same way as (4.22). This chi-squared approximation is generally quite accurate even for small n. If the null hypothesis of no clustering is rejected, we can use the statistic similar to (4.23) to indicate the likely center i of the clustering area with large values of

$$U_i = \frac{1}{C} \sum_{j=1}^{m} \left(\frac{n_i - e_i}{n} \right) \left(\frac{n_j - e_j}{n} \right) a_{ij}$$

which denotes the percentage of the *i*th region's contribution to the significant clustering. Application areas of Tango's index include brain cancer by Fang, Kulldorff, and Gregoris (2004) and prostate cancer by Oliver *et al.* (2006).

Bonetti and Pagano (2005) proposed the use of the interpoint distance distribution in the detection of spatial clustering. Although the development of the test statistic involves some complex elements, the power was shown to be lower than for Tango's index and Kulldorff's spatial scan statistic (Kulldorff, Tango, and Park, 2003). Rogerson (1999) proposed a modified index, called *standardized excess events test* (SEET)

$$R = \sum_{i=1}^{m} \sum_{j=1}^{m} \frac{1}{n} \left(\frac{r_i - p_i}{\sqrt{p_i/n}} \right) \left(\frac{r_j - p_j}{\sqrt{p_j/n}} \right) a_{ij} = \sum_{i=1}^{m} \sum_{j=1}^{m} \frac{1}{n} \left(\frac{n_i - e_i}{\sqrt{e_i}} \right) \left(\frac{n_j - e_j}{\sqrt{e_j}} \right) a_{ij}$$

which is quite similar in form to Walter's adjacency method. However, the power of the modified index with standardized excess events was generally, but not always, less than that of Tango's original index in my limited simulation studies.

Scanning methods

As the first method using scanning of local regional rates, Openshaw *et al.* (1988) developed a Geographical Analysis Machine (GAM) , which is an exploratory tool for searching for potential clusters. The GAM constructs overlapping circles of different radii centered at each grid point defined *a priori*, counts the number of cases and the number of people at risk within the circle, and displays those circles with local incidence proportions exceeding some predefined threshold. However, this GAM has attracted much criticism since it produces a large number of highly correlated overlapped circles. Turnbull *et al.* (1990), on the other hand, proposed a more statistically sound cluster evaluation permutation procedure (CEPP), where, for each region, a window is constructed by absorbing the nearest neighboring regions such that each window contains just a pre-fixed population size R. These windows vary in geographic shape and size but maintain a constant population size at risk so that observed counts are identically distributed. However, these windows of cases and populations overlap; the counts are not independently distributed. The test statistic of CEPP is given by the maximum number of cases (not necessarily integer) in the window. Monte Carlo testing is needed to obtain the p-value for the test statistic.

Besag and Newell (1991) considered windows with a pre-fixed number of cases k rather than a pre-fixed population size. This constant k is considered as the size of the cluster in their method. It was originally designed for quite rare diseases, and thus a typical value of k might be $2, 4, ..., 10$. Each region with nonzero cases is considered in turn as the center of a possible cluster. When considering a particular region, we label it as region 0 and order the remaining regions by their distance to the region 0. We label these regions $1, 2, ..., m-1$ and define

$$v_i = \sum_{j=0}^{i} n_j, \ u_i = \sum_{j=0}^{i} \xi_j$$

so that $v_0 \leq v_1 \leq \cdots$ are the accumulated number of cases in regions $0, 1, ...$ and $u_0 \leq u_1 \leq \cdots$ are the corresponding accumulated size of the population at risk. Now let

$$S = \min\{i : v_i \geq k\}$$

so that the nearest S regions contain the closest k cases. A small observed value of S indicates a cluster centered at region 0. If $s(\geq 1)$ is the observed value of S, then the p-value of each potential cluster is

$$\Pr\{S \leq s\} = 1 - \sum_{t=0}^{k-1} \exp(-u_s Q)(u_s Q)^t / t!, \quad Q = n_+ / \xi_+$$

As a test statistic T_{BN} for overall clustering within the entire study area, Besag and Newell (1991) suggested *the total number of individually significant clusters* ($p < 0.05$, say). The significance of the observed T_{BN} can be determined by Monte Carlo testing. There are several applications of Besag and Newell's method. Besag and Newell themselves illustrate their procedure with data from acute lymphoblastic leukemias in children under the age of 14 years in part of the Mersey Regional Health Authority Districts of England (1975–1985), in which they identified 23 significant clusters. Huillard d'Aignaux *et al.* (2002) applied Besag and Newell's test to detecting spatial clustering in sporadic Creutzfeldt-Jakov disease (CJD) in France during 1992–1998 and identified five clusters that were persistent over a range of values of k.

However, it is quite difficult for users to determine the appropriate cluster size k *a priori*, and thus this test clearly faces multiple testing problems by repeating the test with a number of plausible values of k. Furthermore, it seems questionable whether the *total number of significant clusters* is an appropriate measure as a test statistic because even if we have only one highly significant cluster, the test statistic should give a significant result.

Spatial scan statistics

Kulldorff and Nagarwalla (1995) and Kulldorff (1997) proposed the spatial scan statistic for the Bernoulli model and the Poisson model, which is a spatial version of the scan statistic with a variable window size and is a generalization of CEPP. The spatial scan statistic imposes a circular window $\mathbf{Z}$ on each centroid of the region. In this respect, Kulldorff's spatial scan statistic is also called the *circular spatial scan statistic*. For any of those centroids, the radius of the circle varies from zero to some preset upper limit (as a default, until 50% of the total population is covered). If the window contains the centroid of a region, then that whole region is included in the window. In total, a very large number of different but overlapping circular windows are created, each with a different location and size and each being a potential cluster. Let $\mathbf{Z}_{ik}$, $k = 1, \ldots, K_i$, denote the window composed by the $(k-1)$ nearest neighbors to region i. Then, all the windows to be scanned by the spatial scan statistic are included in the set

$$\mathscr{Z}_1 = \{\mathbf{Z}_{ik} \mid 1 \leq i \leq m,\ 1 \leq k \leq K_i\}$$

Under the alternative hypothesis, there is an elevated risk within some window $\mathbf{Z}$ as compared with outside it:

$$H_0 :\ E(N(\mathbf{Z})) = e(\mathbf{Z}) \quad \text{for all } \mathbf{Z}$$
$$H_1 :\ E(N(\mathbf{Z})) > e(\mathbf{Z}) \quad \text{for some } \mathbf{Z}$$

where $N()$ and $e()$ denote the random number of cases and the null expected number of cases within the specified window, respectively. For each window, it is possible to compute the likelihood of observing the observed number of cases within and outside the window, respectively.

Under the Poisson model described in Section 5.2, the test statistic is the likelihood ratio maximized for $\mathbf{Z}$

$$\lambda = \sup_{\mathbf{Z} \in \mathscr{Z}_1} \left(\frac{n(\mathbf{Z})}{e(\mathbf{Z})}\right)^{n(\mathbf{Z})} \left(\frac{n - n(\mathbf{Z})}{n - e(\mathbf{Z})}\right)^{n - n(\mathbf{Z})} I\left(\frac{n(\mathbf{Z})}{e(\mathbf{Z})} > \frac{n - n(\mathbf{Z})}{n - e(\mathbf{Z})}\right)$$

where $n()$ denotes the observed number of cases within the specified window and $I()$ is the indicator function. The window $\mathbf{Z}^*$ that attains the maximum likelihood is defined as the *most likely cluster* (MLC). To find the distribution of the test statistic under the null hypothesis, Monte Carlo hypothesis testing is required. In practice, we can find significant *secondary clusters* in addition to the most likely significant cluster and order them according to their likelihood ratio test statistic. Especially secondary clusters that do not overlap with the most likely cluster may be of great interest.

Kulldorff's spatial scan statistic has been extended to the ordinal model (Jung, Kulldorff, and Klassen, 2007), the exponential model and the normal model (for these models, see the SaTScan User Guide) and also has been applied to a wide variety of epidemiological studies and to disease surveillance for the detection of disease clusters. This is primarily due to the existence of the freely downloadable software SaTScan (Kulldorff and Information Management Services, 2009), which is easily accessible to a wide range of researchers interested in the detection of clustering. For example, recent application areas include infectious disease (Fang *et al.*, 2006; Polack *et al.*, 2005; Jennings *et al.*, 2005; Bakker *et al.*, 2004), a variety of cancers (Klassen *et al.*, 2006; Pollack *et al.*, 2006; Ozonoff *et al.*, 2005; Han *et al.*, 2004), pediatrics (Viel *et al.*, 2005; Andrade *et al.*, 2004; Boyle *et al.*, 2004), rheumatology (Donnan *et al.*, 2005), variant Creutzfeldt-Jakob disease (Cousens *et al.*, 2001; Huillard d'Aignaux *et al.*, 2002), veterinary medicine (Olea-Popelka *et al.*, 2005; Abriai *et al.*, 2003; Berke and Grosse Beilage 2003) and so on.

However, since it uses a circular window to scan the potential cluster areas, it has difficulty in correctly detecting actual noncircular clusters. To detect arbitrarily shaped clusters that cannot be detected by the circular spatial scan statistic, Patil and Taillie (2004), Duczmal and Assunção (2004), Tango and Takahashi (2005), Assunção *et al.* (2006), and Kulldorff *et al.* (2006) have proposed different spatial scan statistics. Patil and Taillie (2004) used the notion of the "upper level set" to reduce the size of windows to be scanned and proposed the "upper level set scan statistic". However, they do not discuss how to select the level *g*, which defines the upper level set. Duczmal and Assunção (2004), on the other hand, have applied a simulated annealing method in which they try to examine only the most promising windows using a graph-based algorithm to obtain the local maxima of a certain likelihood function over a subset of the collection of all the connected regions. Their method seems to be very complicated, but they do not show any programmable procedure for their method. Tango and Takahashi (2005) called their spatial scan statistic the *flexible spatial scan statistic* in contrast to Kulldorff's *circular spatial scan statistic* and provided FleXScan software (Takahashi, Yokoyama, and Tango, 2009).

The *flexible spatial scan statistic* imposes a flexibly shaped window $\mathbf{Z}$ on each region by connecting its adjacent regions. For any given region i, we create the set of flexibly shaped windows with *length k* consisting of k connected regions including i and let k move from 1 to the preset maximum length of cluster K. To avoid detecting a cluster of *unlikely peculiar shape*, the connected regions are restricted as the subsets of the set of regions i and $(K-1)$ nearest neighbors to the region i. In total, as in the circular spatial scan statistic, a very large number of different but overlapping arbitrarily shaped windows are created. Let $\mathbf{Z}_{ik(j)}$, $j = 1, \ldots, j_{ik}$ denote the jth window, which is a set of k regions connected starting from the region i,

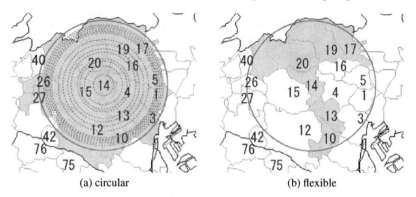

(a) circular   (b) flexible

Fig. 5.3 An example of two different windows: Kulldorff's circular spatial scan statistic and Tango and Takahashi's flexible spatial scan statistic.

where j_{ik} is the number of j satisfying $\mathbf{Z}_{ik(j)} \subseteq \mathbf{Z}_{ik}$ for $k = 1, \ldots, K_i = K$. Then, all the windows to be scanned are included in the set

$$\mathscr{Z}_2 = \{\mathbf{Z}_{ik(j)} \mid 1 \leq i \leq m,\ 1 \leq k \leq K,\ 1 \leq j \leq j_{ik}\}$$

In other words, for any given region i, the circular spatial scan statistic considers K concentric circles, whereas the flexible scan statistic considers K concentric circles plus all the sets of connected regions (including the single region i) whose centroids are located within the Kth largest concentric circle (see Figure 5.3). So, the size of $\mathscr{Z}_2$ is far larger than that of $\mathscr{Z}_1$, which is at most mK. The maximum length K is usually set as 15 or 20 as a default in FleXScan because the method is not currently feasible for cluster sizes larger than 30. The test statistic is of the same form as Kulldorff's test statistic, where $\mathscr{Z}_1$ is replaced by $\mathscr{Z}_2$. Regarding the application of the flexible spatial scan statistic, there is a recent neuro-epidemiological study by Doi *et al.* (2008), who detected a significant cluster of CJD mortality in the northwest region from the base of Mt. Fuji stretching over the two neighboring prefectures of Yamanashi and Shizuoka in Japan.

It should be noted that the spatial scan statistics introduced so far are all based on the maximized likelihood ratio. However, it does not seem to be well-recognized that these likelihood-ratio-based spatial scan statistics tend to detect a MLC much larger than the true cluster by swallowing neighboring regions with nonelevated risk. Tango (2000) shows an example in which Kulldorff's circular spatial scan statistic detected an unrealistically large MLC consisting of 70 regions, much larger than expected from an observed disease map, by absorbing neighboring regions with non-elevated risk of disease occurrence in his simulated data. Furthermore, Tango and Takahashi (2005) have shown interesting but important results in their simulation study in the areas of the Tokyo metropolis and Kanagawa prefecture in Japan, wherein there are $m = 113$ regions that comprise wards, cities, and villages. They applied three spatial scan statistics – Kulldorff's, Duczmal and Assunção's, and Tango

Table 5.1 Regions detected as the most likely cluster by applying three procedures, Kulldorff's circular spatial scan, Tango and Takahashi's flexible spatial scan and Duczmal and Assuncao's spatial scan, to a simulated random sample $n = 235$ from the hot-spot cluster model. In the simulation, the true cluster is assumed to be $\{14, 15, 26, 27\}$ with relative risk 3.0. The maximum length (=number of regions) of the cluster was set to be $K = 15$ (Tango and Takahashi, 2005).

No.	Region no.	Observed no. cases	Expected no. cases	Relative risk (true) $p_i^{\#1}$	One-tailed	Cumulative statistics LLR$^{\#2}$	O/E
1	14	14	3.794	3.69(3)	0.000027	8.3	3.69
2	15	21	6.283	3.34(3)	0.000002	20.1	3.47

Circular's MLC = $\{14, 15\}$, LLR = 20.1, Relative risk = 3.47

No.	Region no.	Observed no. cases	Expected no. cases	Relative risk (true) p_i	One-tailed	LLR	O/E
3	26	6	1.650	3.64(3)	0.004	24.1	3.50
4	27	6	1.964	3.05(3)	0.010	27.3	3.43
5	33	4	1.257	3.18(1)	0.024	29.7	3.41

Flexible's MLC=$\{14, 15, 26, 27, 33\}$, LLR = 29.7, Relative risk = 3.41

No.	Region no.	Observed no. cases	Expected no. cases	Relative risk (true) p_i	One-tailed	LLR	O/E
6	31	3	2.346	1.28(1)	0.313	28.1	3.12
7	48	1	0.696	1.44(1)	0.328	27.8	3.06
8	78	2	1.485	1.35(1)	0.312	27.2	2.93
9	32	5	4.142	1.21(1)	0.318	25.2	2.63
10	77	5	2.109	2.37(1)	0.042	27.2	2.60
11	90	5	2.312	2.16(1)	0.057	29.0	2.57
12	69	3	1.419	2.11(1)	0.114	30.0	2.55
13	24	8	5.534	1.45(1)	0.152	30.0	2.37
14	110	1	0.256	3.91(1)	0.127	30.7	2.38
15	54	1	0.045	22.20(1)	0.022	31.8	2.41

Duczmal Assunção's MLC=$\{14, 15, 26, 27, 33, 31, ..., 54\}$, LLR = 31.8, Relative risk = 2.41

#1: One tailed p_i is defined as (5.21)
#2: LLR = Log likelihood ratio

and Takahashi's – to a simulated disease map consisting of a random sample of $n = 235$ cases by assuming the hot-spot cluster regions $\{14, 15, 26, 27\}$ in which each region's relative risk was set to a constant 3.0 and the cases set to be Poisson distributed and found the following:

- Duczmal and Assunção's (2004) procedure, called a DA scan, detected a quite large and peculiar-shaped MLC that had the largest likelihood ratio among the three MLCs identified by the three spatial scan statistics: Kulldorff's, Duczmal and Assunção's, and Tango and Takahashi's (Table 5.1, Figures 5.4 and 5.5).
- A newly introduced bivariate power distribution (5.22) revealed that the circular spatial scan statistic is shown to have a tendency to detect a cluster much larger than the true cluster assumed in the simulation even when the true cluster is circular.

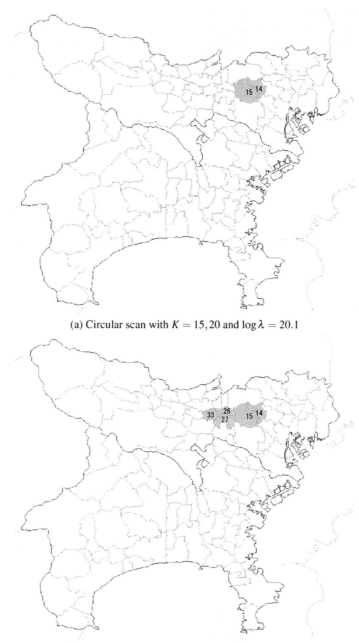

(a) Circular scan with $K = 15, 20$ and $\log \lambda = 20.1$

(b) Flexible scan with $K = 15, 20$ and $\log \lambda = 29.7$

Fig. 5.4 The most likely cluster detected by each of two methods applied to a simulated disease map. (a) Circular scan with $K = 15, 20$ and (b) flexible scan with $K = 15, 20$. The area $C = \{14, 15, 26, 27\}$ is assumed to be the true cluster in the simulation.

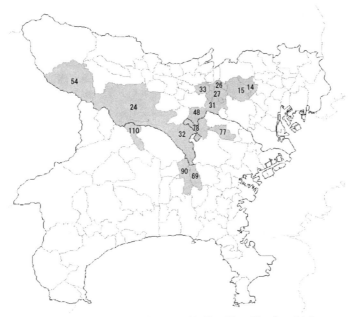

Duczmal and Assunção's scan with $K = 15$ and $\log \lambda = 31.8$

Fig. 5.5 The most likely cluster detected by Duczmal and Assunção's scan with $K = 15$ applied to a simulated disease map. The area $C = \{14, 15, 26, 27\}$ is assumed to be the true cluster in the simulation.

For details of these simulation studies, see Section 5.6. These results cast doubt on the validity of the model selection based on maximizing the ordinary likelihood ratio in general. To cope with this undesirable property of the spatial scan statistics, Kulldorff *et al.* (2006) proposed an elliptic version of the spatial scan statistic based on the likelihood ratio multiplied by the *eccentricity penalty* of the form

$$\lambda = \sup_{\mathbf{Z} \in \mathscr{Z}_3} \left(\frac{n(\mathbf{Z})}{e(\mathbf{Z})} \right)^{n(\mathbf{Z})} \left(\frac{n - n(\mathbf{Z})}{n - e(\mathbf{Z})} \right)^{n - n(\mathbf{Z})} I \left(\frac{n(\mathbf{Z})}{e(\mathbf{Z})} > \frac{n - n(\mathbf{Z})}{n - e(\mathbf{Z})} \right) \left\{ \frac{4s}{(s+1)^2} \right\}^a$$

where s denotes the elliptic window shape defined as the ratio of the length of the longest to the shortest axis of the ellipse and a denotes a penalty tuning parameter. Setting $a = 0$ means "no penalty", but other values of a have no clear interpretable meaning. In SaTScan, we can use either a strong penalty $a = 1$ or a medium penalty $a = 1/2$. This approach is a possible solution but certainly plagued with a large dose of subjectivity and noninterpretability in the penalty parameters. On the other hand, Tango (2008) proposed a spatial scan statistic with a restricted likelihood ratio

$$\lambda = \sup_{\mathbf{Z} \in \mathscr{Z}} \left(\frac{n(\mathbf{Z})}{e(\mathbf{Z})} \right)^{n(\mathbf{Z})} \left(\frac{n - n(\mathbf{Z})}{n - e(\mathbf{Z})} \right)^{n - n(\mathbf{Z})} I \left(\frac{n(\mathbf{Z})}{e(\mathbf{Z})} > \frac{n - n(\mathbf{Z})}{n - e(\mathbf{Z})} \right) \prod_{i \in \mathbf{Z}} I(p_i < \alpha_1)$$

where p_i is the one-tailed *mid-p value* of the test for $H_0 : E(N_i) = \xi_i$ and α_1 is the prespecified screening level for the individual region. In other words, the restricted spatial scan statistic scans only the regions with significantly elevated risk at α_1. This modification can apply to both circular and flexible spatial scan statistics. Tango (2008) illustrates the restricted circular spatial scan statistic with mortality data from cerebrovascular disease in the Tokyo metropolitan area. Tango (2008) recommends $\alpha_1 = 0.2$ as a default via a Monte Carlo simulation study.

5.4 Selected Methods

In this section, we shall describe the details of selected tests for spatial clustering based on regional count data. The selection criteria are (1) *widely known*, (2) *widely used* tests in the literature and (3) free from multiple testing problems.

5.4.1 Tango's Index for Spatial Clustering

Goal: To calculate the clustering index with a measure of closeness between regions and evaluate the significance. A significantly large value would indicate evidence of spatial clustering of the disease under study. This method is also called the *maximized excess events test* (MEET).

Null hypothesis H_0: (5.4)

Alternative hypothesis H_1: not H_0

Test statistic

Let an extension of Tango's index for temporal clustering (4.20) be

$$
\begin{aligned}
C &= (r - p)^t A (r - p) \\
&= \sum_{i=1}^{m} \sum_{j=1}^{m} \left(\frac{n_i - e_i}{n} \right) \left(\frac{n_j - e_j}{n} \right) a_{ij}
\end{aligned}
\tag{5.11}
$$

where $r^t = (n_1, \ldots, n_m)/n$ and

$$
a_{ij} = \exp\left\{ -4 \left(\frac{d_{ij}}{\lambda} \right)^2 \right\}
\tag{5.12}
$$

Then, the test statistic is

$$
P_{\min} = \min_{\lambda} \Pr\{C > c \mid H_0, \lambda\} = \Pr\{C > c \mid H_0, \lambda = \lambda^*\}
\tag{5.13}
$$

where λ varies continuously from a small value near zero upward until λ reaches about one-fourth the maximum distance d_{ij} in the study area,

$$0 < \lambda \le \frac{\max d_{ij}}{4}$$

and λ^* attains the minimum p-values of C. The practical implementation of this procedure is to use "line search" by discretizing λ.

Null distribution

Given λ, the null distribution of C can be asymptotically approximated by the chi-squared distribution

$$\Pr\{C > c \mid H_0\} \approx \Pr\left\{\chi_v^2 > v + \sqrt{2v}\left(\frac{c - E(C)}{\sqrt{\text{Var}(C)}}\right)\right\} \qquad (5.14)$$

where

$$E(C) = n^{-1} tr(\mathbf{AV})$$
$$\text{Var}(C) = 2n^{-2} tr(\mathbf{AV})^2$$
$$v = 8/\{\sqrt{\beta_1(C)}\}^2$$
$$\sqrt{\beta_1(C)} = 2\sqrt{2} tr(\mathbf{AV})^3/\{tr(\mathbf{AV})^2\}^{3/2}$$
$$\mathbf{V} = \sum_{k=1}^{K} \frac{n_{+k}}{n}\{\text{diag}(\mathbf{p}_k) - \mathbf{p}_k \mathbf{p}_k^t\}$$

This chi-squared approximation is generally quite accurate, even for small n. Finally, Monte Carlo hypothesis testing is required to obtain the null distribution of $P_{\min}$ and the Monte Carlo simulated p-value (2.17).

Identifying likely clustering areas

If the null hypothesis of no clustering is rejected, we can use the statistic similar to (4.23) for the case of temporal clustering to indicate the most likely clustering areas i of a clustering area with large values of

$$U_i = \frac{1}{C} \sum_{j=1}^{m} \left(\frac{n_i - e_i}{n}\right)\left(\frac{n_j - e_j}{n}\right) a_{ij} \qquad (5.15)$$

which denote the percentage of the ith region's contribution to the significant clustering. More specifically, we may use the following condition of standardized U_i to suggest the center of the clustering area:

$$Z_i = (U_i - \bar{U})/\text{SD}_U \ge 2.0 \text{ or } 3.0 \qquad (5.16)$$

5.4.2 Kulldorff's Circular Spatial Scan Statistic

Goal: To detect the most likely *circular* hot-spot cluster and secondary clusters, if any, within the study area divided into several regions and evaluate its (their) statistical significance. The finding that the most likely cluster is significant would suggest evidence for the existence of a localized circular cluster within the study area.

Null hypothesis and alternative hypothesis
The null hypothesis H_0 given by (5.4) and the alternative hypothesis H_1 are expressed as

$$H_0: E(N(\mathbf{Z})) = e(\mathbf{Z}) \quad \text{for all } \mathbf{Z}$$

$$(5.17)$$

$$H_1: E(N(\mathbf{Z})) > e(\mathbf{Z}), \quad \text{for some } \mathbf{Z}$$

where $\mathbf{Z}$ denotes a *circular window* imposed on the centroid of a region and $N(\mathbf{Z})$ and $e(\mathbf{Z})$ denote the random number of cases and the *conditional* null expected number of cases within the specified window $\mathbf{Z}$, respectively. Under the alternative hypothesis, it is assumed that there is a hot spot cluster or an elevated risk within some window $\mathbf{Z}$ as compared with outside it.

Test statistic

$$\lambda = \sup_{\mathbf{Z} \in \mathcal{Z}_1} \left(\frac{n(\mathbf{Z})}{e(\mathbf{Z})} \right)^{n(\mathbf{Z})} \left(\frac{n - n(\mathbf{Z})}{n - e(\mathbf{Z})} \right)^{n - n(\mathbf{Z})} I \left(\frac{n(\mathbf{Z})}{e(\mathbf{Z})} > \frac{n - n(\mathbf{Z})}{n - e(\mathbf{Z})} \right) \quad (5.18)$$

where window $\mathbf{Z}$ to be scanned by the spatial scan statistic is included in the set

$$\mathcal{Z}_1 = \{ \mathbf{Z}_{ik} \mid 1 \le i \le m, \ 1 \le k \le K_i \}$$

where $\mathbf{Z}_{ik}$, $k = 1, \ldots, K_i$, denotes the window composed by the $(k-1)$ nearest neighbors to region i. The value of K_i depends on the starting region i so that the radius of the circle varies from zero upward until 50% of the total population is covered. The window $\mathbf{Z}^*$ that attains the maximum likelihood is defined as the *most likely cluster* (MLC). If the most likely cluster is significant, then we can search for significant *secondary clusters* that do not overlap with the most likely cluster, if any, and order them according to their likelihood ratio test statistic.

Null distribution

Monte Carlo hypothesis testing is required to obtain the null distribution of λ and the Monte Carlo simulated p-value (2.17). The p-value of a secondary cluster is obtained by comparing its likelihood with the null distribution of λ.

Software

SaTScan: http://www.satscan.org/

5.4.3 Tango and Takahashi's Flexible Spatial Scan Statistic

Goal: To detect the most likely *flexibly shaped* hot-spot cluster and secondary clusters, if any, within the study area divided into several regions and evaluate its (their) statistical significance. The finding that the most likely cluster is significant would suggest evidence for the existence of a localized cluster within the study area.
Null hypothesis and alternative hypothesis: (5.17)

Test statistic

$$\lambda = \sup_{\mathbf{Z} \in \mathscr{Z}_2} \left(\frac{n(\mathbf{Z})}{e(\mathbf{Z})} \right)^{n(\mathbf{Z})} \left(\frac{n - n(\mathbf{Z})}{n - e(\mathbf{Z})} \right)^{n - n(\mathbf{Z})} I \left(\frac{n(\mathbf{Z})}{e(\mathbf{Z})} > \frac{n - n(\mathbf{Z})}{n - e(\mathbf{Z})} \right) \quad (5.19)$$

where $\mathbf{Z}$ denotes a *flexibly shaped window* to be scanned by the spatial scan statistic are included in the set

$$\mathscr{Z}_2 = \{ \mathbf{Z}_{ik(j)} \mid 1 \le i \le m, \ 1 \le k \le K, \ 1 \le j \le j_{ik} \}$$

where $\mathbf{Z}_{ik(j)}$, $j = 1, \ldots, j_{ik}$, denotes the jth window that is a set of k regions connected starting from the region i and j_{ik} is the number of j satisfying $\mathbf{Z}_{ik(j)} \subseteq \mathbf{Z}_{ik}$ for $k = 1, \ldots, K_i = K$. The cluster size or the maximum length K of the cluster is usually set to 15 or 20. The window $\mathbf{Z}^*$ that attains the maximum likelihood is defined as the *most likely cluster* (MLC). If the most likely cluster is significant, then we can search for significant *secondary clusters* that do not overlap with the most likely cluster, if any, and order them according to their likelihood ratio test statistic.

Null distribution

Monte Carlo hypothesis testing is required to obtain the null distribution of λ and the Monte Carlo simulated p-value (2.17). The p-value of a secondary cluster is obtained by comparing its likelihood with the null distribution of λ.

Software

FleXScan: http://www.niph.go.jp/soshiki/gijutsu/download/flexscan/index.html

5.4.4 Tango's Spatial Scan Statistic with Restricted Likelihood Ratio

Goal: To detect the most likely cluster consisting of connected regions with elevated risk only and secondary clusters, if any, within the study area divided into several regions and evaluate its (their) statistical significance. The finding that the most likely cluster is significant would suggest evidence for the existence of a localized cluster consisting of regions with elevated risk.

Null hypothesis and alternative hypothesis: (5.17)

Test statistic

$$\lambda = \sup_{\mathbf{Z} \in \mathscr{Z}} \left(\frac{n(\mathbf{Z})}{e(\mathbf{Z})} \right)^{n(\mathbf{Z})} \left(\frac{n - n(\mathbf{Z})}{n - e(\mathbf{Z})} \right)^{n - n(\mathbf{Z})} I \left(\frac{n(\mathbf{Z})}{e(\mathbf{Z})} > \frac{n - n(\mathbf{Z})}{n - e(\mathbf{Z})} \right) \prod_{i \in \mathbf{Z}} I(p_i < \alpha_1)$$

$$(5.20)$$

where the set of windows $\mathscr{Z}$ can be either Kulldorff's circular set $\mathscr{Z}_1$ or Tango and Takahashi's flexible set $\mathscr{Z}_2$, p_i is the one-tailed *mid-p value* of the test for H_0 : $E(N_i) = e_i$,

$$p_i = \Pr\{N_i \geq n_i + 1 \mid N_i \sim \text{Poisson}(\xi_i)\} + \frac{1}{2} \Pr\{N_i = n_i \mid N_i \sim \text{Poisson}(\xi_i)\} \quad (5.21)$$

and α_1 is the prespecified screening level for the individual region. The window $\mathbf{Z}^*$ that attains the maximum likelihood is defined as the *most likely cluster* (MLC). If the most likely cluster is significant, then we can search for significant *secondary clusters* that do not overlap with the most likely cluster, if any, and order them according to their likelihood ratio test statistic.

Choice of α_1

The choice of α_1 is totally up to users. When users do not have any idea how to choose the value of α_1, Tango (2008) provides a guideline regarding the choice of α_1 for a restricted likelihood ratio test of the nominal α level of 0.05:

1. $\alpha_1 = 0.10 \sim 0.20$ to detect small clusters with a sharp increase in risk,
2. $\alpha_1 = 0.20 \sim 0.30$ to detect small to middle-sized clusters with a moderate increase in risk,
3. $\alpha_1 = 0.30 \sim 0.40$ to detect larger clusters with a slight increase in risk.

Tango (2008) recommends $\alpha_1 = 0.20$ as a default.

Null distribution

Monte Carlo hypothesis testing is required to obtain the null distribution of λ and the Monte Carlo simulated p-value (2.17). The p-value of a secondary cluster is obtained by comparing its likelihood with the null distribution of λ.

Software

FleXScan: http://www.niph.go.jp/soshiki/gijutsu/download/flexscan/index.html

5.5 Illustration with Real Data

5.5.1 Japanese Gallbladder Cancer Mortality Data

As an illustration, we shall apply three tests, (1) spatial clustering index, 2) circular spatial scan statistic, and (3) flexible spatial scan statistic, to the data for mortality from gallbladder cancer (male, 1996–2000) in the area of three adjacent prefectures (Niigata, Fukushima, and Yamagata) in Japan. The total observed number of deaths for five years was 665 in this area, with $m = 246$ regions (cities and villages). The variability of the number of deaths per region is 0 (25th percentile), 1 (median), 3 (75th percentile), 60 (maximum), which means that mortality from gallbladder cancer is rare. Before applying these three tests for spatial clustering, let us recall the disease maps of relative risks estimated in Chapter 3.

Figure 3.4 shows the choropleth map of SMRs for gallbladder cancer (male). No clear spatial pattern emerges from this map. SMRs are commonly used in disease mapping but are very unstable in the sense that they can yield large changes in estimates with relatively small changes in the expected number of cases. When studying a rare disease and small areas, the most extreme SMRs may be based on only a few cases. To overcome the drawbacks of the SMRs in disease mapping, Bayesian approaches have been considered. One approach is an empirical Bayes approach that adopts the Poisson-gamma model but the numbers of observed deaths in each region are assumed to be mutually independent. Figure 3.6 shows the choropleth map of EBSMRs for gallbladder cancer (male). We can observe high risks in the three areas (the dark areas) located at the coastline extending from west to northeast and observe lower risks (the shaded areas) in the southeast. One disadvantage of the Poisson-gamma model is its inability to deal with spatial correlation; i.e., the relative risks for adjacent regions could be similar. The CAR model proposed by Besag, York and Mollie (1991) takes spatial autocorrelation into account. We applied the CAR model using WinBUGS and showed the estimates for the relative risk of gallbladder cancer mortality (male) in Figure 3.10. The choropleth maps in Figure 3.6 and Figure 3.10 present a similar geographical pattern for the relative risks, but the estimates of the CAR model provide more smoothed variations in relative risk and indicate high risk in two coastal areas. It should be noted, however, that all the Bayesian 95% credible intervals of these estimates of relative risk include 1.0 due to the small number of deaths per region, although the disease map highlights the two high-risk areas (the dark areas).

Tango's index for spatial clustering
Next, we shall apply Tango's index for spatial clustering using the R function
TangoS.index. (Appendix). The input data required for this program are in two different files:

1. Case file ("dat" in the R program):
   Format: < region ID > < Observed No. cases > < Expected No. cases >
2. Coordinate file: ("geo" in the R program)
   Format: < region ID > < y-coordinate > < x-coordinate > or
           < region ID > < Latitude > < Longitude >

Regarding a sequence of values of cluster size λ ("lam" in the R program), we considered 21 values of λ $(0.1, 5, 10, 15, ...95, 100)$ since $\max d_{ij}/4 = 311.8/4 = 78.0$.

An example using the R function TangoS.index

```
> geo< −scan("gallblad.geo",list(id=0, y=0, x=0))
> dat< −scan("gallblad.dat",list(id=0, d=0, e=0))
> lam< −c(0.1, (1:20)*5 )
> Nrep< −999;
> out< −TangoS.index(dat, geo, lam, Nrep)
> out$p.value
[1] 0.001
> out$id[out$stdcont>=2.0]
[1] 15201 7204 6204 7203 15306 15307
> signif(out$stdcont[out$stdcont>=2.0], 3)
[1] 10.10 6.87 5.50 3.38 2.31 2.14
> signif(out$smr[out$stdcont>=2.0], 3)
[1] 1.31 0.63 1.92 0.65 4.27 3.94
```

In this application, we consider the test statistic

$$P_{\min} = \min_{\lambda \in \{0.1, 5, 10, ..., 100\}} \Pr\{C > c \mid H_0, \lambda\}$$

and obtained $P_{\min} = 0.00004$ at $\lambda^* = 45$. The adjusted p-value of $P_{\min}$ was $1/(999 + 1) = 0.001$ by Monte Carlo testing with 999 replicates. Figures 5.6–5.8 show three figures that are outputs from the R program above. Figure 5.6 shows the profile p-value of Tango's index C and the optimal $\lambda^* = 45$, which attains the minimum of the

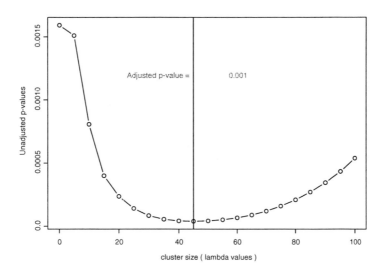

Fig. 5.6 The profile p-value of Tango's index C applied to gallbladder cancer mortality (male) in three adjacent prefectures, Niigata, Fukushima, and Yamagata, in Japan (1996–2000). The vertical line denotes the optimal λ^* that attains the minimum of the profile p-value.

profile p-value. Figure 5.7 shows the geographical heterogeneity of population size in 246 regions. Figure 5.8 shows the observed number of deaths in these regions, and circles are drawn only for the regions whose observed-to-expected ratio, n_i/e_i, is statistically significantly larger than 1.0 at $\alpha = 0.05$ or

$$Q_i = \Pr\{N_i \leq n_i \mid N_i \sim \text{Poisson}(e_i)\}.$$

The area is set inversely proportional to the tail probability Q_i, suggesting that many circles are clustered around two coastline areas highlighted by the CAR model (Figure 3.10). Figure 5.9 shows the percentage contribution to C due to each of 246 regions, and the corresponding region code is also shown. The top six regions (satisfying $Z_i > 2.0$) with large contributions to the significant clustering are shown in Table 5.2. Three coastal regions (15201, 15306 and 15307) and a northern coastal region (6204) are indicated in Figure 5.10. It should be noted that another northern coastal region (6461) ranks seventh, with $Z_i = 1.88$.

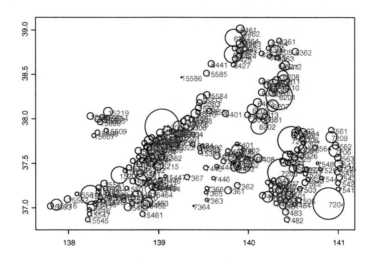

Fig. 5.7 Locations of 246 regions (indicated by region code) comprising cities and villages in the area of three adjacent prefectures, Niigata, Fukushima, and Yamagata, in Japan. The center of a circle is the location of the population centroid of the corresponding region, and the area is set proportional to the population size.

Table 5.2 The top six regions (satisfying $Z_i > 2.0$) that made a large contribution to the significant spatial clustering of gallbladder cancer mortality (male) detected by Tango's index C in the area of three adjacent prefectures, Niigata, Fukushima, and Yamagata, in Japan (1996–2000).

Rank	Region code	Observed number	Expected number	SMR	Percentage contribution	Std Percentage contribution	Risk type
	i	n_i	e_i		U_i	Z_i	
1	15201	60	45.869	1.308	17.269	10.181	High
2	7204	24	38.082	0.630	11.617	6.769	Low
3	6204	22	11.459	1.920	9.422	5.443	High
4	7203	18	27.694	0.650	5.973	3.361	Low
5	15306	5	1.171	4.269	4.311	2.357	High
6	15307	5	1.269	3.939	4.041	2.194	High

Circular spatial scan statistic

Next, we shall apply Kulldorff's circular spatial scan statistic using the software SaTScan (2009 version). Details of data files and their formats required for SaTScan are omitted here (check with the SaTScan user's guide). The following is a part of the output.

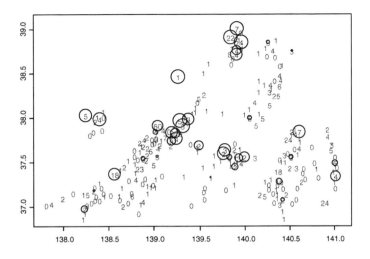

Fig. 5.8 The observed number of deaths from gallbladder cancer (male) for each of 246 regions in the area of three adjacent prefectures, Niigata, Fukushima, and Yamagata, in Japan (1996–2000). Circles are drawn only for the regions whose observed-to-expected ratios are statistically significantly larger than 1.0 at $\alpha = 0.05$. The area is set proportional to the tail probability.

Output from SaTScan program for purely spatial analysis

MOST LIKELY CLUSTER

1.Location IDs included.: 6462, 6461, 6464, 6204, 6463, 6422,
                          6421, 6426, 6423, 6424
Coordinates / radius..: (38.968333 N, 139.945833 E) / 28.28 km
Population............: 239671
Number of cases.......: 46
Expected cases........: 23.97
Annual cases / 100000.: 19.2
Observed / expected...: 1.919
Relative risk.........: 1.988
Log likelihood ratio..: 8.340324
Monte Carlo rank......: 22/1000
P-value..............: 0.022

SECONDARY CLUSTERS
2.Location IDs included.: 15221, 15306, 15307, 15302, 15303,
                          15323, 15304, 15206, 15324, 15309,
                          15308, 15301, 15201, 15207, 15218,
                          15347
Coordinates / radius..: (37.913333 N, 139.222222 E) / 19.59 km
Population............: 867828
Number of cases.......: 124
Expected cases........: 86.78
Annual cases / 100000.: 14.3
Observed / expected...: 1.429
Relative risk.........: 1.527
Log likelihood ratio..: 8.259382
Monte Carlo rank......: 23/1000
P-value..............: 0.023

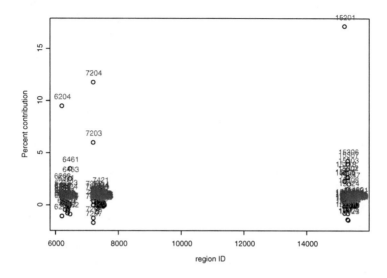

Fig. 5.9 Percentage contribution to the value of Tango's index C for each of 246 regions in the application to gallbladder cancer mortality (male) in the area of three adjacent prefectures, Niigata, Fukushima, and Yamagata, in Japan (1996–2000). The number shown in the plot denotes the region code.

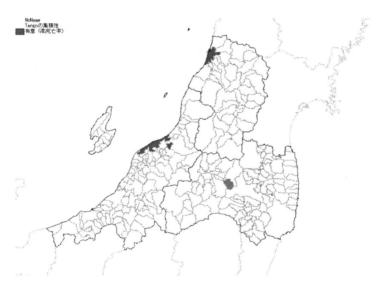

Fig. 5.10 Two high-risk coastal areas detected by Tango's index C for spatial clustering in the application to gallbladder cancer mortality (male) in the area of three adjacent prefectures, Niigata, Fukushima, and Yamagata, in Japan (1996–2000).

In Figure 5.11(a), the most likely cluster and the secondary cluster are indicated. These two high-risk areas roughly correspond with those estimated by the CAR model (Figure 3.10).

Flexible spatial scan statistic

Next, we shall show application of Tango and Takahashi's flexible spatial scan statistic using the software FleXScan (2009 version). Here also, we omit the details of the data files for FleXScan. The following is a part of the output.

Output from FleXScan program for purely spatial analysis

MOST LIKELY CLUSTER

1.Census areas included .: 06204, 06364, 06421, 06423, 06424,
                          06461, 06463, 06464
Maximum distance.......: 36.5586 km (areas: 06204 to 06364)
Number of cases ....: 46   (21.0453 expected)
Overall relative risk .: 2.18576
Log likelihood ratio ..: 11.5056
Monte Carlo rank ......: 22/1000
P-value ....: 0.022

SECONDARY CLUSTERS

2.Census areas included .: 15201, 15206, 15218, 15301, 15302,
                          15303, 15306, 15307, 15308, 15324,
                          15347, 15384
Maximum distance.......: 37.7298 km (areas: 15201 to 15384)
Number of cases ....: 112   (72.195 expected)
Overall relative risk .: 1.55135
Log likelihood ratio ..: 10.7447
Monte Carlo rank ......: 41/1000
P-value ....: 0.041

In Figure 5.11(b), the most likely cluster and the secondary cluster are indicated. These two high risk areas also roughly correspond to those estimated by the CAR model (Figure 3.10). The most likely cluster and the secondary cluster detected by the flexible spatial scan statistic are very similar to, but slightly different from, those of the circular spatial scan statistic.

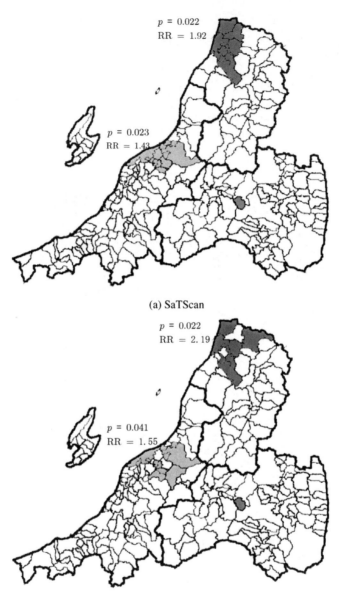

Fig. 5.11 The most likely cluster (thick) and the secondary cluster (thin) of gallbladder cancer mortality (male) detected by (a) SaTScan (upper) and (b) FleXScan (lower) in the area of three adjacent prefectures, Niigata, Fukushima, and Yamagata, in Japan (1996–2000)

Tango's spatial scan statistic with restricted likelihood ratio
 The two spatial scan statistics detected similar but slightly different MLCs and secondary clusters, which agree well with two coastal high-risk areas estimated by EBSMRs and CAR models. However, the regional number of deaths from gallbladder cancer in this area is very small and thus let's examine these detected regions in more detail. The observed number of deaths, expected number of deaths, SMR, and one-tailed p-value (5.21) are shown in Table 5.3. Surprisingly, SaTScan's significant MLC includes one region (6462) with 0 cases, its significant secondary cluster includes two regions (15323, 15304) with 0 cases, and FleXScan's significant secondary cluster includes one region (15384) with 0 cases. Furthermore, significant MLCs or secondary clusters include regions where the observed number of deaths is almost equal to the expected number. These regions are 6464, 6422, 6421, 6426, 15221, 15309, and 15207. In other words, about half of the regions included in the significant MLCs or secondary clusters do not have any elevated risk. Therefore, a question naturally arises in our mind: Are these significant MLCs and secondary clusters really "*clusters of regions with significantly elevated risk*"? These phenomena exactly match those described in the previous section; i.e., "*...these likelihood ratio based spatial scan statistics tend to detect the most likely cluster much larger than the true cluster by swallowing neighboring regions with non-elevated risk*". Then, we shall apply Tango's spatial scan statistic with the restricted likelihood ratio by using four different values of α's; i.e., $\alpha_1 = 0.2, 0.3, 0.4, 0.5$. The results are as follows.

	Circular scan			Flexible scan		
α_1	MLC	SMR	p-value	MLC	SMR	p-value
0.20	15218, 15301, 15303	17/7.73 =2.20	0.461	6204, 6461	29/13.88=2.09	0.245
0.30	15206, 15306, 15307 15308	24/11.91=2.02	0.271	7402, 7404, 7406 7407, 7421, 7422 7424, 7441, 7442 7443	24/10.23=2.34	0.240
0.40	15206, 15306, 15307 15308	24/11.91=2.02	0.285	7402, 7404, 7406 7407, 7421, 7422 7424, 7441, 7442 7443	24/10.23=2.34	0.285
0.50	15206, 15306, 15307 15308	24/11.91=2.02	0.305	6204, 6364, 6421 6423, 6424, 6461 6463, 6464	46/21.05=2.19	0.006

 None of these results are statistically significant except that for the flexible scan with $\alpha_1 = 0.5$, which detected the same significant MLC as the flexible scan with the ordinary likelihood ratio. Therefore, unless investigators accept that the regions with $p_i = 0.40 \sim 0.50$ can be included in the MLC, we might consider that we could not find any single significant MLC or hot-spot cluster of gallbladder cancer mortality.

Table 5.3 Regions detected as the most likely cluster and the secondary cluster by Kulldorff's circular spatial scan and Tango and Takahashi's flexible spatial scan applied to gallbladder cancer (male) in three adjacent prefectures, Niigata, Fukushima, and Yamagata, in Japan, 1996–2000.

No.	Region code	Observed no. cases	Expected no. cases	SMR	One-tailed $p_i^{\#1}$	Spatial scan statistic SaTScan	FleXScan
Most likely cluster							
1	6462	0	1.074	0.000	0.8291	*	
2	6461	7	2.419	2.894	0.0078	*	*
3	6464	1	0.977	1.023	0.4398	*	*
4	6204	22	11.459	1.920	0.0027	*	*
5	6463	4	0.801	4.991	0.0053	*	*
6	6422	2	2.226	0.898	0.5180	*	
7	6421	1	0.984	1.016	0.4424	*	*
8	6426	1	1.092	0.916	0.4812	*	
9	6423	4	1.614	2.479	0.0526	*	*
10	6424	4	1.321	3.029	0.0283	*	*
11	6364	3	1.470	2.041	0.1228		*

SaTScan's MLC : LLR = 8.34, Relative risk = 1.988
FleXScan's MLC : LLR = 11.51, Relative risk = 2.186

No.	Region code	Observed no. cases	Expected no. cases	SMR	One-tailed $p_i^{\#1}$	SaTScan	FleXScan
Secondary cluster							
1	15221	4	4.255	0.940	0.5178	*	
2	15306	5	1.171	4.269	0.0042	*	*
3	15307	5	1.269	3.939	0.0058	*	*
4	15302	3	0.883	3.398	0.0363	*	*
5	15303	5	2.193	2.280	0.0481	*	*
6	15323	0	1.101	0.000	0.8337	*	
7	15304	0	1.212	0.000	0.8512	*	
8	15206	11	8.589	1.281	0.2028	*	*
9	15324	4	3.055	1.310	0.2795	*	*
10	15309	1	0.986	1.014	0.4429	*	
11	15308	3	0.881	3.407	0.0361	*	*
12	15301	4	1.263	3.167	0.0250	*	*
13	15201	60	45.869	1.308	0.0222	*	*
14	15207	7	7.795	0.898	0.5895	*	
15	15218	8	4.272	1.872	0.0498	*	*
16	15347	4	1.989	2.011	0.0963	*	*
17	15384	0	0.762	0.000	0.7665		*

SaTScan's MLC : LLR = 8.26, Relative risk = 1.527
FleXScan's MLC : LLR = 10.74, Relative risk = 1.551

#1: One-tailed p_i is defined as (5.21)

5.5.2 New York Incident Leukemia Cases

The data considered here are 592 incident leukemia cases from 1978 to 1982 for each of 790 census tracts among 1,057,673 people at risk in an eight-county region of upstate New York. This data set was originally reported and analyzed by Waller *et al.* (1992, 1994). For a detailed description of this data set, see Waller and Gotway (2004). Some of the leukemia cases could not be georeferenced to the corresponding census tract, and the location is known only within a few neighboring census tracts. These cases were then allocated in proportion to the population in each census tract. Therefore, most of the case counts have noninteger values. In this situation, we cannot use SaTScan due to noninteger case counts. However, Kulldorff and Nagarwalla (1995) illustrated their method with this data set and thus I shall cite their result. Furthermore, as we have no information about the adjacency between census tracts we cannot apply FleXScan. So, we shall apply Tango's index only.

Tango's index for spatial clustering

The geographical locations of five cities, Binghamton, Cortland, Syracuse, Auburn, and Ithaca, and 592 leukemia cases are shown in Figure 5.2, in which circles are drawn only for the census tracts whose observed-to-expected ratio is statistically significantly larger than 1.0 at $\alpha = 0.05$. The radius is set inversely proportional to the tail probability. We can observe that census tracts with statistically significantly elevated risk are located near these major cities.

In this application, we have $\max d_{ij}/4 = 160/4 = 40$, and we considered 20 values of $\lambda = 2, 4, 6, ..., 38, 40$,

$$P_{\min} = \min_{\lambda \in \{2,4,...,40\}} \Pr\{C > c \mid H_0, \lambda\}$$

We obtained $P_{\min} = 0.0000003$ at $\lambda^* = 6$ km. Since this p-value is the lowest value of 999 Monte Carlo p-values, the adjusted p-value is $p = 1/(999+1) = 0.001$ using Monte Carlo testing with 999 replicates (Figure 5.12).

Four clusters were detected from the top 19 census tracts that made large contributions (i.e., standardized $U_i \geq 3.0$) to significant clustering, $p = 0.001$. The radius of the circle drawn in Figure 5.13 is set proportional to the size of the contribution, U_i. As a matter of fact, there were 11 inactive hazardous waste sites containing TCE (trichloroethylene) in this area. Exposure to TCE was a motivating concern of the epidemiological study. Locations of inactive hazardous waste sites, S1,..., S11, and four clusters, A, B, C, D, of incident leukemia cases are shown in Figure 5.14. It seems interesting that cluster A includes four TCE sites, S1, S2, S3, and S4, cluster B is located near the sites S7 and S11, and cluster D includes the site S5.

Kulldorff's circular spatial scan statistic

In this chapter, we have described the Poisson models only. To this data set, Kulldorff and Nagarwalla (1995) applied a Bernouilli model, not a Poisson model, where we have cases and noncases represented by 0 or 1 variable and cases and noncases constitute the population as a whole. They identified the two significant clusters; i.e., the most likely cluster ($p = 0.005$) is located in the same area as cluster A, and the secondary cluster ($p = 0.027$) is in the same area as cluster B, shown in Figure 5.13.

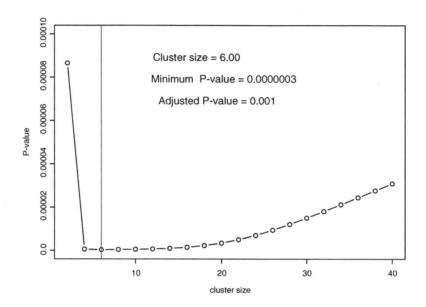

Fig. 5.12 The profile *p*-value of Tango's index for spatial clustering C applied to 592 incident leukemia cases.

5.6 Power Comparison

Power

There have been several papers comparing tests for spatial randomness, but there have been few simulation studies for comparing three or more tests. Among other things, Kulldorff, Tango, and Park (2003) created a collection of 1,220,000 simulated benchmark data, generated under 51 different clustering models, to evaluate the power of different test statistics for various types of clusters. These data sets are based on the 1990 female population in the 245 counties and county equivalents in the northeastern United States. Each county is represented by a centroid coordinate. Using these benchmark data, Kulldorff, Tango, and Park (2003) and Song and Kulldorff (2003) conducted intensive power comparison studies among several tests that have been published. These studies have shown that

- Kulldorff's circular spatial scan statistic is shown to be the most powerful for detecting localized clusters,
- Tango's index is most powerful for general clustering throughout the study area, and the

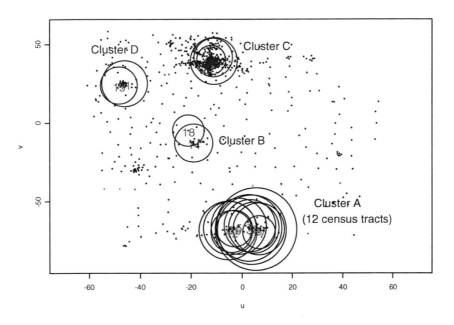

Fig. 5.13 Four clusters, A, B, C, and D, of incident leukemia cases detected by Tango's index in an eight-county region of upstate New York (1978–1982), These clusters were constructed using the top 19 census tracts that made large contribution to the significant clustering ($p = 0.001$). u and v denote coordinates of the centroid of each region. Dot "." denotes the location of each of 790 census tracts. The radius of each circle drawn is set proportional to the size of the contribution, U_i.

- Besag-Newell test has the best power for mixed or multiple clusters, but its strength is very sensitive to the choice of cluster size k.

Bivariate power distribution

It should be noted, however, that the power estimates provided reflect only the "power to reject the null hypothesis for whatever reason" and that the probability of both rejecting the null hypothesis and detecting the true cluster correctly is a different matter. Especially, the ultimate goal of spatial scan statistics is to identify the localized clusters correctly, if any, and so a *high usual power* is not a sufficient condition for a *good* spatial scan statistic. To investigate *the performance* of spatial scan statistics, Tango and Takahashi (2005) proposed a new bivariate power distribution $P(l,s)$ based upon Monte Carlo simulation that is the probability that the significant most likely cluster has length $l (\geq 1)$ and includes s regions within the true cluster with length s^*

$$P(l,s) = \frac{\#\{\text{significant MLC has length } l \text{ and includes } s \text{ true regions}\}}{\#\{\text{trials for each simulation}\}} \quad (5.22)$$

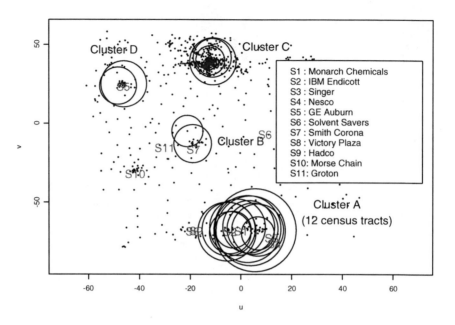

Fig. 5.14 Locations of inactive hazardous waste sites, S1,..., S11, and four clusters, A, B, C, and D, of incident leukemia cases detected by Tango's index in an eight-county region of upstate New York (1978–1982)

where $1 \leq l$ and $0 \leq s \leq \min\{l, s^*\}$. In particular, we are interested in the power around the point $(l = s^*, s = s^*)$ and $P(s^*, s^*)$, the probability of exact detection. Then, the usual power is defined as the sum of $P(l, s)$:

$$P(+, +) = \sum_{l=1}^{l_{\max}} \sum_{s=0}^{\min\{l, s^*\}} P(l, s) = 1 - P(0, 0) \qquad (5.23)$$

where $l_{\max}$ denotes the maximum length l observed in the simulation and $P(0, 0)$ denotes the probability that the spatial scan statistic cannot detect any clusters. Based on this bivariate power distribution, Tango and Takahashi (2005) compared the performance of the circular spatial scan statistic with that of the flexible spatial scan statistic. As an entire study population, they used $m = 113$ regions comprising the wards, cities, and villages in the area of Tokyo metropolis and Kanagawa prefecture in Japan (Figure 5.15). The variability of regional populations for $m = 113$ regions is 25th percentile = 56,704, median= 142,320 and 75th percentile = 200,936.

On this map, they considered several types of hot-spot clusters. Two of them are

- $A = \{14, 15, 20\}$ (circular cluster; $s^* = 3$)

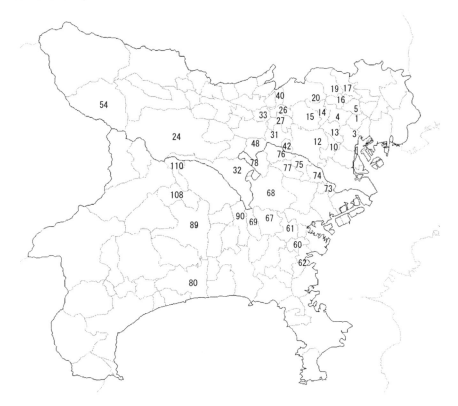

Fig. 5.15 The 113 regions that comprise wards, cities, and villages in the areas of Tokyo metropolis and Kanagawa prefecture in Japan. The region number used in the text is also indicated. In particular, the region numbers of two hot-spot clusters considered in this paper are $\mathbf{A} = \{14, 15, 20\}$ (circular cluster; $s^* = 3$) and $\mathbf{C} = \{14, 15, 26, 27\}$ (noncircular cluster; $s^* = 4$).

- $\mathbf{C} = \{14, 15, 26, 27\}$ (noncircular cluster; $s^* = 4$)

where the relative risk within the hot-spot cluster was set to 3.0. The powers are calculated for tests of nominal α levels of 0.05 and for the expected total number of cases (200) under the null hypothesis, which are based on Monte Carlo simulation using Poisson random numbers. For making power comparisons to a certain extent fair, they chose a common maximum length $K = 15$ although Kulldorff's circular scan statistic can vary the radius until 50% of the total population is covered. For each simulation, 1000 trials were carried out. The resultant power distributions $P(l, s) \times 1000$ are reproduced in Tables 5.4 and 5.5 for each of the cluster models in the form of cross tables classified by l ("*length*" in tables) and s ("*include*" in tables), respectively.

Both tests have high "usual power" for the circular cluster $\mathbf{A}$ (Table 5.4), while Tango and Takahashi's scan statistic has higher power for the noncircular cluster $\mathbf{C}$ (Table 5.5). Table 5.4 shows that Kulldorff's scan statistic detects the cir-

Table 5.4 Comparison of the bivariate power distribution $P(l,s) \times 1000$ between the circular spatial scan statistic and the flexible spatial scan statistic for the hot-spot cluster A={14, 15, 20}. The nominal α-level is set as 0.05, and 1000 trials are carried out (Tango and Takahashi, 2005).

Circular ($K = 15$)

Length l	Include s hot-spot regions 0	1	2	3	Total
1	0	0			0
2	1	0	0		1
3	0	0	0	738	738
4	0	0	0	134	134
5	0	0	0	39	39
6	0	0	0	12	12
7	0	0	0	9	9
8	0	0	0	1	1
9	0	0	2	3	5
10	0	0	0	2	2
11	0	0	0	4	4
12	0	0	0	12	12
13	0	0	0	14	14
14	0	0	0	3	3
15	0	0	0	6	6
Total	1	0	2	977	980

Usual power = 0.980

Flexible ($K = 15$)

Length l	Include s hot-spot regions 0	1	2	3	Total
1	0	0			0
2	0	0	0		0
3	0	0	0	142	142
4	0	0	0	116	116
5	0	0	0	137	137
6	0	0	0	149	149
7	0	0	0	165	165
8	0	0	0	131	131
9	0	0	0	84	84
10	0	0	0	27	27
11	0	0	0	11	11
12	0	0	0	2	2
13	0	0	0	0	0
14	0	0	0	0	0
15	0	0	0	0	0
Total	0	0	0	964	964

Usual power = 0.964

cular cluster **A** considerably accurately with power $P(3,3) = 738/1000$, while Table 5.5 shows that it exhibits zero power $P(4,4) = 0/1000$ for detecting the noncircular cluster **C** accurately. On the other hand, Tango and Takahashi's scan statistic does not exhibit such high power for identifying the clusters accurately: $P(3,3) = 142/1000$ for the cluster **A** and $P(4,4) = 138/1000$ for the cluster **C**. However, the power distribution appears to be concentrated in a relatively narrow range of the length l on the line $s = s^*$, thereby indicating that the observed significant MLC contains the true cluster with a considerably high probability. In particular, for the cluster **C** with length $s^* = 4$, the marginal power of Tango and Takahashi's scan statistic $P(+,s^*) = 850/1000$ and its conditional marginal power $P(+,s^*)/P(+,+) = 850/890$ are much higher than those of Kulldorff's scan statistic, $P(+,s^*) = 254/1000$ and $P(+,s^*)/P(+,+) = 254/801$, respectively. Furthermore, Kulldorff's scan statistic exhibits a greater tendency to detect a larger cluster than the true cluster as compared with that of Tango and Takahashi. For example, the probability that the length of MLC for the cluster **C** ($s^* = 4$) is greater than or equal to 12 is 213/1000, compared with 2/1000 for Tango and Takahashi's scan statistic. This tendency is shown even in the circular cluster **A**, where the same probabilities are 35/1000 vs. 2/1000.

In summary, the Monte Carlo simulation study using the bivariate power distribution reveals the following findings:

Table 5.5 Comparison of the bivariate power distribution $P(l,s) \times 1000$ between the circular spatial scan statistic and the flexible spatial scan statistic for the hot-spot cluster $\mathbf{C}=\{14, 15, 26, 27\}$. The nominal α-level is set as 0.05, and 1000 trials are carried out (Tango and Takahashi, 2005).

Circular ($K = 15$)							Flexible ($K = 15$)					
Length l	Include s hot-spot regions					Total	Length l	Include s hot-spot regions				Total
	0	1	2	3	4			0 1 2 3			4	
1	1	0				1	1	0 0				0
2	0	0	351			351	2	0 0 0				0
3	2	0	4	0		6	3	0 0 0	0			0
4	0	0	3	0	0	3	4	0 0 0	0		138	138
5	2	0	2	0	0	4	5	0 0 0	3		147	150
6	1	0	0	0	0	1	6	1 0 0	2		200	203
7	0	0	0	81	0	81	7	0 1 0	4		147	152
8	0	0	10	18	38	66	8	0 0 2	9		107	118
9	0	0	2	0	26	28	9	0 0 0	10		71	81
10	0	0	0	29	3	32	10	1 0 2	5		28	36
11	0	0	1	13	1	15	11	0 0 0	0		10	10
12	0	0	2	4	60	66	12	0 0 0	0		2	2
13	0	0	0	5	62	67	13	0 0 0	0		0	0
14	0	0	0	10	27	37	14	0 0 0	0		0	0
15	0	0	0	6	37	43	15	0 0 0	0		0	0
Total	6	0	375	166	254	801	Total	2 1 4	33		850	890

Usual power = 0.801   Usual power = 0.890

- The circular spatial scan statistic shows a high level of accuracy in detecting circular clusters exactly and reasonably good power for including some hot-spot regions in the most likely cluster.
- The flexible spatial scan statistic exhibits no such high power regarding exact identification of clusters, but the support of the power distribution is shown to be concentrated in a relatively narrow range of length l on the line $s = s^*$, indicating that an observed significant most likely cluster contains the true cluster with quite high probability.
- The circular spatial scan statistic, on the other hand, is shown to have zero power for detecting exactly noncircular clusters that cannot be captured by any circular window.
- The circular spatial scan statistic is also shown to have a tendency to detect a larger cluster than the true cluster assumed in the simulation, even for the case where the true cluster is circular.

To summarize the bivariate power distribution, Takahashi and Tango (2006) proposed an *extended power* of cluster detection tests that includes the usual power as a special case.

Spatial scan statistic tends to detect larger clusters

Tango (2008) conducted a similar power comparison between Kulldorff's circular spatial scan statistic and Tango's restricted circular spatial scan statistic using the bivariate power distribution where the radius of the circle varies from zero upward until 50% of the total population at risk is covered. Table 5.6 shows the result for the hot-spot circular cluster $\mathbf{A} = \{14, 15, 20\}$ with relative risk 3.0 and $n = 200$. This table shows a good characteristic of the restricted circular spatial scan statistic. Namely, it could detect the hot-spot circular cluster $\mathbf{A}$ with length $s^* = 3$ considerably accurately with powers $P(3,3) = 0.834$, 0.864, 0.767, 0.755, 0.748 for $\alpha_1 = 0.05$, 0.10, 0.20, 0.30, 0.40, respectively. When we also evaluate the power of detecting the true cluster plus one additional region, its power is also high without reference to the value of α_1: $P(3,3) + P(4,3) = 0.882$, 0.976, 0.957, 0.918, 0.906 for $\alpha_1 = 0.05$, 0.10, 0.20, 0.30, 0.40, respectively. The maximum length of the MLCs among all the results was only $l = 8$. On the other hand, Kulldorff's circular spatial scan statistic also had relatively high powers such as $P(3,3) = 0.672$ and $P(3,3) + P(4,3) = 0.819$. However, the estimated bivariate power distribution had a long tail to the right on the line $s = 3$, and the maximum length was 47. The usual power of the restricted circular spatial scan statistic was larger than that of Kulldorff's circular spatial scan statistic except for the case of $\alpha_1 = 0.05$.

Tables 5.7 and 5.8 show the results for the hot-spot circular cluster

$$\mathbf{C} = \{1, 4, 5, 12, 13, 14, 15, 16, 19, 20\}$$

with smaller relative risk 2.0 and $n = 200$. In this instance, Kulldorff's circular spatial scan statistic was expected to detect changes in a larger area that may not be obvious from each region individually and had high usual power, 0.807, with the exact detection probability $P(10, 10) = 0.323$. However, the support of the estimated bivariate power distribution was again scattered over a broad area on the plane $\{(l, s) : l \geq s, l = 1, 2, ..., 51, s = 0, 4, 8, 9, 10\}$ by swallowing up many additional regions. In contrast, Table 5.8 shows that the support of the restricted circular spatial scan statistic was distributed in a relatively confined area on the plane (l, s). However, the results with $\alpha_1 = 0.05$ and 0.10 were miserable; i.e., their usual powers were quite low, 0.039 and 0.161, respectively. As the value of α_1 increased, the usual power increased to 0.548, 0.741, and 0.744 for $\alpha_1 = 0.20$, 0.30, and 0.40, respectively. Although the probability of detecting the cluster exactly was zero without reference to the value of α_1 chosen, the restricted circular spatial scan statistic was shown to have a high probability of pinpointing eight or nine regions out of $s^* = 10$ regions: $P(8,8) + P(9,9) = 0.713$, 0.703 for $\alpha_1 = 0.30$, 0.40, respectively.

These results suggest that:

- For larger clusters with smaller relative risk, the usual power of Kulldorff's circular spatial scan statistic was higher than that of the restricted circular spatial scan statistic.
- Kulldorff's MLCs tended to be much larger than the true cluster in order to try to include the true cluster within the MLC.
- The restricted circular spatial scan statistic had higher powers of detecting a part of the true cluster when $\alpha_1 = 0.30$ or 0.40.

Table 5.6 Estimated bivariate power distributions $P(l,s) \times 1000$ of Kulldorff's circular spatial scan statistic and the restricted circular spatial scan statistic for the hot-spot circular cluster $\mathbf{A} = \{14, 15, 20\}$ with relative risk 3.0 and $n = 200$. The nominal α-level is set as 0.05, and 1000 trials are carried out. In this comparison, the radius of the circle varies from zero upward until 50% of the total population at risk is covered (Tango, 2008).

Kulldorff's circular scan

Length l	Include s hot-spot regions 0 1 2	3
1	1 0	
2	0 0 0	
3	0 0 0	672
4	0 0 0	147
5	0 0 0	38
6	0 0 0	26
7	0 0 0	8
8	0 0 0	3
9	0 0 0	1
10	0 0 0	3
11	0 0 0	3
12	0 0 0	13
13	0 0 0	15
14	0 0 0	4
15	0 0 0	2
16–20	0 0 0	13
21–25	0 0 0	6
26–30	0 0 0	1
31–35	0 0 0	2
36–40	0 0 0	3
41–45	0 0 0	1
46–47	0 0 0	1
Total	1 0 0	962

Usual power = 0.963

Restricted circular scan

α_1	Length l	Include s hot-spot regions 0 1 2	3	Usual power
0.05	1	1 0		0.885
	2	1 0 0		
	3	0 0 0	834	
	4	0 0 0	48	
	5	0 0 0	1	
0.10	1	1 0		0.984
	2	0 0 0		
	3	1 0 0	864	
	4	0 0 0	112	
	5	0 0 0	5	
	6	0 0 0	1	
0.20	1	1 0		0.978
	2	0 0 0		
	3	1 0 0	767	
	4	0 0 0	190	
	5	0 0 0	16	
	6	0 0 0	3	
0.30	1	1 0		0.978
	2	0 0 0		
	3	1 0 0	755	
	4	0 0 0	163	
	5	0 0 0	42	
	6	0 0 0	16	
0.40	1	1 0		0.978
	2	0 0 0		
	3	0 0 0	748	
	4	0 0 0	158	
	5	0 0 0	45	
	6	0 0 0	22	
	7–8	0 0 0	4	

This finding may suggest that if other spatial scan statistics for detecting arbitrary-shaped clusters adopted the proposed likelihood ratio, their performance might be expected to improve.

Judging from my experience using both circular and flexible spatial scan statistics based on the ordinary likelihood ratio or the restricted likelihood ratio, circular and flexible spatial scan statistics are complementary tools that each have their strengths and should be used together irrespective of the type of likelihood ratio.

Table 5.7 Estimated bivariate power distributions $P(l,s) \times 1000$ of Kulldorff's circular spatial scan statistic for the hot-spot circular cluster $\mathbf{C} = \{1,4,5,12,13,14,15,16,19,20\}$ with relative risk $\theta_C = (2.0,2.0,2.0,2.0,2.0,2.0,2.0,2.0,2.0,2.0)$ and $n = 200$. The nominal α-level is set as 0.05, and 1000 trials are carried out. In this comparison, the radius of the circle varies from zero upward until 50% of the total population at risk is covered (Tango, 2008).

| | Kulldorff's circular scan | | | | | | | | | | |
| Length l | Include s hot-spot regions | | | | | | | | | | |
	0	1	2	3	4	5	6	7	8	9	10
1	5	0									
2	0	0									
3	0	0	0	0							
4	0	0	0	0	0						
5	0	0	0	0	0	0					
6	0	0	0	0	1	0	0				
7	0	0	0	0	0	0	0	0			
8	0	0	0	0	0	0	0	0	0		
9	0	0	0	0	0	0	0	0	0	0	
10	0	0	0	0	0	0	0	0	0	0	323
11	0	0	0	0	0	0	0	0	9	0	56
12	0	0	0	0	0	0	0	0	12	0	23
13	0	0	0	0	0	0	0	0	5	4	97
14	0	0	0	0	0	0	0	0	5	1	16
15	0	0	0	0	0	0	0	0	0	3	32
16	0	0	0	0	0	0	0	0	0	5	19
17	0	0	0	0	0	0	0	0	0	1	28
18	0	0	0	0	0	0	0	0	0	0	28
19	0	0	0	0	0	0	0	0	0	0	12
20	0	0	0	0	0	0	0	0	0	0	9
21–25	0	0	0	0	0	0	0	0	0	0	38
26–30	0	0	0	0	0	0	0	0	13	0	21
31–35	0	0	0	0	0	0	0	0	4	0	11
36–40	0	0	0	0	0	0	0	0	1	6	8
41–45	0	0	0	0	0	0	0	0	0	0	5
46–50	0	0	0	0	0	0	0	0	1	0	4
51	0	0	0	0	0	0	0	0	0	0	1
Total	5	0	0	0	1	0	0	0	50	20	731

Usual power = 0.807

Notwithstanding, the development of a spatial scan statistic with high accuracy and precision will be an open problem worth future work.

Table 5.8 Estimated bivariate power distributions $P(l,s) \times 1000$ of the restricted circular spatial scan statistic for the hot-spot circular cluster $\mathbf{C} = \{1,4,5,12,13,14,15,16,19,20\}$ with relative risk $\theta_C = (2.0,2.0,2.0,2.0,2.0,2.0,2.0,2.0,2.0,2.0)$ and $n = 200$. The nominal α-level is set as 0.05 and 1000 trials are carried out. In this comparison, the radius of the circle varies from zero upward until 50% of the total population at risk is covered (Tango, 2008).

		Restricted circular scan											Usual power
α_1	Length l	Include s hot-spot regions											
		0	1	2	3	4	5	6	7	8	9	10	
0.05	1	10	0										0.019
	2	6	0	0									
	3	1	0	0	0								
	4	0	0	0	0	2							
0.10	1	8	0										0.161
	2	7	0	0									
	3	2	0	0	0								
	4	0	0	0	0	110							
	5	0	0	0	0	0	33						
	6	0	0	0	0	0	1	0					
0.20	1–4	12	0	0	0	0							0.548
	5	0	0	0	0	0	403						
	6	0	0	0	0	0	58	0					
	7	0	0	0	0	0	0	3	0				
	8	0	0	0	0	0	0	0	0	0			
	9	0	0	0	0	0	0	0	0	0	71		
	10–12	0	0	0	0	0	0	0	0	0	1	0	
0.30	1–5	9	0	0	0	0	0						0.741
	6	0	0	0	0	1	0	0					
	7	0	0	0	0	0	0	3	0				
	8	0	0	0	0	0	0	0	0	138			
	9	0	0	0	0	0	0	0	2	0	575		
	10	0	0	0	0	0	0	0	1	0	0	0	
	11–12	0	0	0	0	0	0	0	0	9	3	0	
0.40	1–5	9	0	0	0	0	0						0.744
	6	0	0	0	0	1	0	0					
	7	0	0	0	0	0	0	2	0				
	8	0	0	0	0	0	0	0	0	135			
	9	0	0	0	0	0	0	0	6	0	568		
	10	0	0	0	0	0	0	0	1	0	0	0	
	11	0	0	0	0	0	0	0	0	8	0	0	
	12	0	0	0	0	0	0	0	0	4	7	0	
	13–14	0	0	0	0	0	0	0	0	3	0	0	

Chapter 6
General Tests for Spatial Clustering : Case-Control Point Data

We shall consider here the problem of detecting disease clustering in space based on case-control location data, which is illustrated by the following two examples with Tables 6.1 and 6.2.

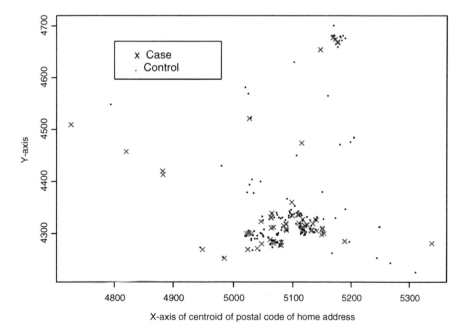

Fig. 6.1 Locations of 62 cases of childhood leukemia and lymphoma and 141 controls between 1974 and 1986 in the North Humberside area (data from Cuzick and Edwards, 1990).

T. Tango, *Statistical Methods for Disease Clustering*,
Statistics for Biology and Health, DOI 10.1007/978-1-4419-1572-6_6,
© Springer Science+Business Media, LLC 2010

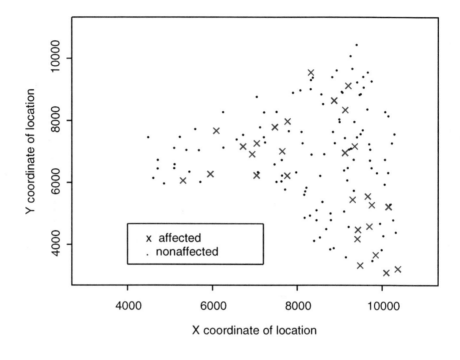

Fig. 6.2 Locations of 143 early medieval grave sites. Locations indicated "x" denote those grave sites where the person shows evidence of a particular tooth defect (data from Waller and Gotway, 2004).

Example 1

Figure 6.1 shows the locations of 62 cases of childhood leukemia and lymphoma diagnosed in North Humberside between 1974 and 1986 and 141 controls selected at random from entries in the birth register for January 7 or June 7 for each of the years 1974–1986. Centroids of postal codes of home addresses were used to obtain grid references for mapping these data where the unit of measurement is 100 m. Does this figure suggest any pattern of clustering of cases?

Example 2

Figure 6.2 shows the data on 143 early medieval grave sites (Waller and Gotway, 2004). The anthropologists and archaeologists conducted an investigation of an early medieval burial ground in Neresheim, Germany, to examine whether the particular culture tended to place grave sites according to family unit. They used inherited features in the teeth of excavated skeletons to mark a subset of sites. This figure includes 30 grave sites where skeletons have affected teeth (graves of "affected individuals") and 113 where they did not. The research question here is whether there is any clustering of affected sites.

6.1 Data

Throughout this chapter, it is assumed that:

1. n_0 cases are observed in the study region, and a set of n_1 controls are selected at random from all individuals at risk in the study region using, for example, electoral lists, census information, or birth registers, so that the control could be a representative sample of the study region with the same distribution as the case regarding important confounders such as sex and age.
2. Let $(z_1, \ldots, z_n)$, $n = n_0 + n_1$, denote the locations of cases or controls in the combined sample where the indices have been randomly permuted so that the z_i's contain no information about group membership.
3. For $i = 1, \ldots, n$, define

$$\delta_i = \begin{cases} 1 \text{ if } z_i \text{ is a case} \\ 0 \text{ if } z_i \text{ is a control} \end{cases} \tag{6.1}$$

where $\sum_{i=1}^{n} \delta_i = n_0$.
4. The Euclidean distance between two points z_i and z_j is defined as d_{ij}.

In order to adjust for confounders such as sex and age that may produce an uninteresting apparent clustering, we should adopt either stratification of the cases and population from which the control sample is taken or matching one or more controls to each case.

6.2 Null Hypothesis vs. Alternative Hypothesis

Intuitively, the null hypothesis of no clustering can be stated as

$$H_0 : \text{ cases and controls are independently and randomly sampled}$$
$$\text{from the same population} \tag{6.2}$$

Statistically, the null hypothesis of no clustering can be expressed as

> H_0 : the location of cases follows an inhomogeneous Poisson
>
> process with spatially varying intensity $\lambda(z)$ (6.3)

where the intensity is a function of the (age- snd sex-specific) population density. However, the population density is generally unknown or is difficult to compute on a local scale. Therefore, to avoid the difficulties in estimating the intensity function, Cuzick and Edwards (1990) proposed selecting a random sample of controls from the population at risk so that the null hypothesis of no clustering can be stated as

> H_0 : the observed n_0 case series is a random sample from the entire
>
> sample of size $n_0 + n_1$ combining cases and controls   (6.4)

The null hypothesis (6.4) is called the *random labeling hypothesis*, in which we can make a permutational inference conditional on the observed locations of cases and controls. Under the random labeling hypothesis, we have

$$\text{Pr}\{\text{an arbitrary } z_i \text{ is a case} \mid \text{random labeling hypothesis}\} = \frac{n_0}{n} \quad (6.5)$$

which suggests that the random labeling hypothesis (6.4) does not need to make explicit reference to an underlying inhomogeneous Poisson process of cases or controls. In other words, the superposition of cases and controls constitutes a realization of a stationary and isotropic homogeneous Poisson process with a constant intensity where we can use the K-function (2.2).

6.3 Historical Overview of Methods

(It should be noted that there are several other proposed methods not mentioned here. Furthermore, readers who are not interested in the history can skip this section.)

The first statistical method that employs a sample of case-control data is Cuzick and Edwards' test (1990), which has often been used in the literature (for example, see Alexander *et al.*, 1992; Childs *et al.*, 1998; Dockerty, Sharples, and Borman, 1999; Doherr *et al.*, 2002; Perez *et al.*, 2002; Carpenter *et al.*, 2006). Although Alt and Vach (1991) independently developed an identical procedure, this approach is referred to as the Cuzick and Edwards test here because they provided detailed inferential procedures. Although Cuzick and Edwards considered several nearest neighbor test statistics, their primary test statistic is defined as the sum, over all cases, of the number of each case's k nearest neighbors that also are cases, which is given by the quadratic form:

$$T_k = \sum_{i=1}^{n} \sum_{j=1}^{n} \delta_i \delta_j a_{ij}(k)$$

where

$$a_{ij}(k) = \begin{cases} 1, & \text{if } z_j \text{ is among the } k \text{ nearest neighbors to } z_i \\ 0, & \text{otherwise} \end{cases}$$

When cases are clustered, T_k will be large since nearest neighbors to a case tend to be other cases. The approach is epidemiologically rational in that it accounts for not only geographical variation in population density but also confounders via the judicious selection of controls. However, Tango (2007) noted the following inferential problems inherent in Cuzick and Edwards' test:

- This approach also suffers from multiple testing if the test is repeated multiple times with different values of k. Cuzick and Edwards applied their procedure to a data set on the locations of cases of childhood leukemia and lymphoma diagnosed in North Humberside between 1974 and 1986, an example highlighting the importance of choosing the correct value of k. In a simulation study, Song and Kulldorff (2003) showed that the power of this test is very sensitive to the choice of the unknown number k.
- Cuzick and Edwards showed that their test statistic has an asymptotically normal distribution, but this seems to be questionable for moderately large sample sizes.
- If the clustering process is related to the model of "decline in risk with distance," which has often been used to examine environmental excess risks around putative sources, their test could produce an *apparent significant clustering* since their test statistic gives equal weight to all k nearest neighbors irrespective of whether the distance to the nearest neighbors is large or small.

To adjust for multiple testing, Cuzick and Edwards proposed a linear combination of several different preselected T_k's. It seems to me, however, that the interpretation of "linear combination" is not so easy. Tango (2007) proposed a class of tests with quadratic forms that includes Cuzick and Edwards' test statistic as a special case

$$T(\theta) = \sum_{i=1}^{n} \sum_{j=1}^{n} \delta_i \delta_j a_{ij}(\theta)$$

where $a_{ij}(\theta)$ could be any measure of the closeness between two points z_i and z_j with $a_{ii}(\theta) = 0$ for all $i = 1, \ldots, n$ and θ denotes an unknown parameter related to cluster size. Tango (2007) considers the *double exponential clinal model*

$$a_{ij}(\theta) = \begin{cases} \exp\{-4(\frac{d_{ij}}{\theta})^2\}, & \text{if } i \neq j \\ 0, & \text{if } i = j \end{cases}$$

where θ is a predetermined scale of clusters such that any pair of cases far apart beyond the distance θ cannot be considered as a cluster. The double exponential clinal model with $a_{ii}(\theta) = 1$, shown in equation (5.12), has been used in Tango's (2000) index for spatial disease clustering based on regional count data. However, the two test statistics are essentially the same because $T(\theta \mid a_{ii}(\theta) = 1) = T(\theta \mid a_{ii}(\theta) = 0) + n_0$. Depending on the situation, we can use other measures of closeness; for example, a *hot-spot model*:

$$a_{ij}(\theta) = \begin{cases} 1, \text{ if } d_{ij} \leq \theta \ (i \neq j) \\ 0, \text{ otherwise} \end{cases}$$

Tango (2007) further proposed (i) a central chi-squared distribution with degrees of freedom adjusted by skewness as a better asymptotic distribution of the test statistic, (ii) the *minimum of the profile p-value of the test statistic for the parameter* as an integrated test statistic not only to adjust for multiple testing but also to estimate the optimal cluster size, and (iii) a statistic to search for the areas or cases that have large contributions to significant clustering.

Rogerson (2006) also proposed a simple statistic to search for the clustering areas by dividing the study region into n_0 subregions by letting each control location be the center of a *Thiessen polygon* so that locations inside the polygon are closer to its center than to any other center. Then, the candidate for the clustering area is simply the polygon with a large number of cases that are located inside the polygon. Jacquez (1994) proposed an extension to Cuzick and Edwards' approach when case and control locations are not known exactly; for example, when cases and controls are assigned to centroids of zip codes.

On the other hand, Diggle and Chetwynd (1991) developed an approach to the assessment of spatial clustering based on the second-order properties of the stationary and isotropic spatial point process, namely the K-function (2.2). Although the main purpose of Diggle and Chetwynd's approach was to estimate the nature and physical scale of clustering effects rather than test for their existence, they noted that the formal significance test is also available using Monte Carlo hypothesis testing. Their test statistic is the difference between the K-function for cases and that for controls,

$$D(s) = K_{\text{case}}(s) - K_{\text{control}}(s)$$

However, this test statistic is not the usual form for testing if cases tend to show spatial clustering after being adjusted for the heterogeneity of spatial patterns of controls. To see this, consider the estimates of the K-function without the edge correction term (which is enough for disease clustering; see Section 2.2), which is given by

$$\hat{K}_{\text{case}}(s) = \frac{|A|}{n_0(n_0 - 1)} \sum_{i=1}^{n} \sum_{j=1, j \neq i}^{n} \delta_i \delta_j I(d_{ij} \leq s)$$

$$\hat{K}_{\text{control}}(s) = \frac{|A|}{n_1(n_1 - 1)} \sum_{i=1}^{n} \sum_{j=1, j \neq i}^{n} (1 - \delta_i)(1 - \delta_j) I(d_{ij} \leq s)$$

These estimates clearly indicate that the K-function for cases without the edge correction term is equivalent to Tango's test statistic stated above with *a hot-spot* measure of closeness. Now, take another look at the difference $\hat{D}(s)$, which is decomposed into two parts

$$\hat{D}(s) = [\hat{K}_{\text{case}}(s) - E_{H_0}\{\hat{K}_{\text{case}}(s)\}] - [\hat{K}_{\text{control}}(s) - E_{H_0}\{\hat{K}_{\text{control}}(s)\}]$$

where

$$E_{H_0}\{\hat{K}_{\text{case}}(s)\} = E_{H_0}\{\hat{K}_{\text{control}}(s)\} = \frac{|A|}{n(n-1)} \sum_{i=1}^{n} \sum_{j=1, j\neq i}^{n} I(d_{ij} \leq s)$$

The first part of $\hat{D}(s)$ should be a test statistic for spatial clustering of cases after adjusting for heterogeneity of spatial pattern of controls and the second part is a test statistic for spatial clustering of controls after adjusting for heterogeneity of cases. That is, a positive value of $\hat{D}(s)$ suggests a spatial clustering of cases that is larger than the spatial clustering of controls. Therefore, Diggle and Chetwynd's test statistic should be used when we would like to *compare the degree of spatial clustering of cases with that of controls*. Although there are several examples of Diggle and Chetwynd's procedure in the literature (for example, see O'Brien et al., 2000; Broman et al., 2006), it does not seem to me that users understand well the above-stated characteristic of Diggle and Chetwynd's procedure.

So far, we have implicitly described the methods related to *global clustering tests* designed for evaluating whether cases tend to come in groups or are located close to each other no matter when and where they occur. When we are interested in detecting localized clusters and evaluating their significance, called *cluster detection tests*, we can use the circular spatial scan statistic proposed by Kulldorff and Nagarwalla (1995) and Kulldorff (1997) that was already described for the case of regional count data in Chapter 5. It should be noted, however, that with case-control point data we express the likelihood ratio in terms of the Bernoulli distribution rather than the Poisson distribution for regional count data.

6.4 Selected Methods

In this section, we shall describe the details of tests for spatial clustering based on case-control location data that are selected in terms of *widely known and/or widely used tests* in the literature.

6.4.1 Cuzick and Edwards' Test

Goal: To calculate the sum, over all cases, of the number of each case's k nearest neighbors that are also cases and evaluate the significance. A significantly large number would indicate evidence of spatial clustering of the disease under study;

i.e., cases tend to be located close to each other no matter where they occur.

Null hypothesis H_0: (6.4)

Alternative hypothesis H_1: not H_0

Test statistic

For a predefined value of cluster size k, the test statistic is defined as the sum, over all cases, of the number of each case's k nearest neighbors that also are cases, called the k nearest neighbors method

$$T_k = \sum_{i=1}^{n} \sum_{j=1}^{n} \delta_i \delta_j a_{ij}(k) \tag{6.6}$$

where

$$a_{ij}(k) = \begin{cases} 1, & \text{if } z_j \text{ is among the } k \text{ nearest neighbors to } z_i \\ 0, & \text{otherwise} \end{cases} \tag{6.7}$$

When ties exist in the data, namely when there exist three cases z_i, z_{j_1}, z_{j_2} such that $d_{ij_1} = d_{ij_2}$, the $a_{ij_1}(k)$ and $a_{ij_2}(k)$ values are no longer always zero or unity. In such a case, Cuzick and Edwards assigned a_{ij} the probability that a point is a k nearest neighbor to some other point. For example, if $k = 4$ and the third, fourth, and fifth nearest neighbors $\{j_1, j_2, j_3\}$ are tied, then we put

$$a_{ij}(3) = 1/3, \ a_{ij}(4) = 2/3, \ a_{ij}(5) = 1, \quad \text{for } j \in \{j_1, j_2, j_3\}$$

The approach has been extended by Jacquez (1994) to allow upper- and lower-bound test statistics to be calculated.

Null distribution

The null distribution of the test statistic is approximated by a normal distribution

$$Z_k = \frac{T_k - E(T_k)}{\sqrt{\text{Var}(T_k)}} \sim N(0,1) \tag{6.8}$$

where

$$p_j = \prod_{l=0}^{j} \frac{n_0 - l}{n - l} \tag{6.9}$$

$$N_s = \sum_i \sum_j a_{ij}(k) a_{ji}(k) \tag{6.10}$$

$$N_t = \sum_i \sum_j \sum_{l \neq i} a_{ij}(k) a_{lj}(k) \tag{6.11}$$

$$E(T_k) = p_1 k n \tag{6.12}$$

$$\text{Var}(T_k) = (kn + N_s) p_1 (1 - p_1) + \{(3k^2 - k)n + N_t - 2N_s\}(p_2 - p_1^2)$$
$$- \{k^2(n^2 - 3n) + N_s - N_t\}(p_1^2 - p_3) \tag{6.13}$$

The normal approximation above is generally good even for small n. However, Monte Carlo hypothesis testing is required under the random labeling hypothesis to obtain a more accurate null distribution of Z_k and the Monte Carlo simulated p-value (2.17).

Combined test statistic to adjust for multiple testing
The power of the test statistic T_k is known to be very sensitive to the choice of the unknown cluster size k, and repeating the analysis using a different k is very useful to give an idea of what value of k is likely to be best. However, formal significance testing requires some adjustment for multiple testing. To do this, Cuzick and Edwards considered a linear combination of the T_k

$$T_{\text{comb}} = \mathbf{1}' \boldsymbol{\Sigma}^{-1/2} \boldsymbol{T} \tag{6.14}$$

where $\boldsymbol{T} = (T_{k_1}, ..., T_{k_m})'$ for some subset of size m of the T_k, $\boldsymbol{\Sigma} = \text{Cov}(T_{k_1}, ..., T_{k_m})$, $\mathbf{1} = (1, ..., 1)$, and

$$
\begin{aligned}
\text{Cov}(T_k, T_l) &= \{kn + N_s(k,l)\} p_1 (1 - p_1) \\
&\quad + \{(3kl - k)n + N_t(k,l) - 2N_s(k,l)\}(p_2 - p_1^2) \\
&\quad - \{kl(n^2 - 3n) + N_s(k,l) - N_t(k,l)\}(p_1^2 - p_3)
\end{aligned} \tag{6.15}
$$

$$N_s(k,l) = \sum_i \sum_j a_{ij}(k) a_{ji}(l) \tag{6.16}$$

$$N_t(k,l) = \sum_i \sum_j \sum_{m \neq i} a_{ij}(k) a_{mj}(l) \tag{6.17}$$

Under the null hypothesis, it is approximated that

$$Z_{\text{comb}} = \frac{T_{\text{comb}} - E(T_{\text{comb}})}{\sqrt{\text{Var}(T_{\text{comb}})}} \sim N(0, 1) \tag{6.18}$$

where

$$E(T_{\text{comb}}) = np_1 \sum_j \sum_k j \left((j,k) \text{ element of the matrix } \boldsymbol{\Sigma}^{-1/2} \right)$$

$$\text{Var}(T_{\text{comb}}) = m$$

However, Monte Carlo hypothesis testing is required under the random labelling hypothesis to obtain a more accurate null distribution of Z_{comb} and the Monte Carlo simulated p-value (2.17).

6.4.2 Tango's Index for Spatial Clustering

Goal: To calculate a generalized version of Cuzick and Edwards' test statistic and evaluate the significance. A significantly large value would indicate evidence of spatial clustering of the disease under study; i.e., cases tend to be located close to each other no matter where they occur.

Null hypothesis H_0: (6.4)

Alternative hypothesis H_1: not H_0

Test statistic

Let $T(\theta)$ denotes a generalized test statistic of Cuzick and Edwards's T_k:

$$T(\theta) = \sum_{i=1}^{n} \sum_{j=1}^{n} \delta_i \delta_j a_{ij}(\theta) = \boldsymbol{\delta}' A(\theta) \boldsymbol{\delta} \qquad (6.19)$$

where $A = (a_{ij}(\theta))$ could be any matrix of a measure of the closeness between two points z_i and z_j with $a_{ii} = 0$ for all $i = 1, \ldots, n$, θ denotes an unknown parameter related to cluster size, and $\boldsymbol{\delta} = (\delta_1, \ldots, \delta_n)^t$. Then, Tango's test statistic is

$$P_{\min} = \min_{\theta_L \le \theta \le \theta_U} \Pr\{T(\theta) > t(\theta) \mid H_0, \theta\}$$
$$= \Pr\{T(\theta^*) > t(\theta^*) \mid H_0, \theta = \theta^*\} \qquad (6.20)$$

where $t(\theta)$ is the observed test statistic at θ, θ_L and θ_U denote the user-defined lower bound and upper bound for θ, respectively, and θ^* attains the minimum p-values of $T(\theta)$.

Selection of measure of closeness

In the test statistic (6.20), $a_{ij}(\theta)$ could be any measure of closeness between two points. Tango (2007) especially considered the following two cases:

1. $k(= \theta)$ nearest neighbors model:
   When we adopt $a_{ij}(k)$ of (6.6) as a measure of closeness, then the test statistic $T(\theta) = T_k$ is Cuzick and Edwards (1990) k nearest neighors test statistic. As $a_{ij}(k)$ defined by (6.7) is not symmetric and the later general development of the distribution under the null hypothesis requires a symmetric property for $a_{ij}(k)$, we shall replace $a_{ij}(k)$ by

$$a_{ij}(k) \leftarrow \frac{a_{ij}(k) + a_{ji}(k)}{2} \qquad (6.21)$$

   It should be noted that the transformation does not affect the Cuzick and Edwards test statistic.

2. A double exponential clinal model

$$a_{ij}(\theta) = \begin{cases} \exp\{-4(\frac{d_{ij}}{\theta})^2\}, & \text{if } i \neq j \\ 0, & \text{if } i = j \end{cases} \qquad (6.22)$$

where θ is a predetermined scale of clustering such that any pair of cases far apart beyond the distance θ cannot be considered a cluster. The double exponential clinal model with $a_{ii}(\theta) = 1$, shown in equation (5.12), has been used in Tango's (2000) index for spatial disease clustering based on regional count data.

Needless to say, depending on the situation, we can use other a_{ij}'s $(i \neq j)$ that are nondecreasing functions of distance; for example, another exponential model

$$a_{ij}(\theta) = \begin{cases} \exp\{-\frac{d_{ij}}{\theta}\} & \text{if } i \neq j \\ 0 & \text{if } i = j \end{cases} \tag{6.23}$$

and a hot-spot model:

$$a_{ij}(\theta) = \begin{cases} 1, \text{ if } d_{ij} \leq \theta \ (i \neq j) \\ 0, \text{ otherwise} \end{cases} \tag{6.24}$$

The exponential model (6.23) seems in general to be reasonable, but interpretation of the scale parameter θ is not so clear compared with that of the double exponential model.

Null distribution of $T(\theta)$

As in the case of Tango's index for temporal clustering (4.20) and that for spatial clustering (5.11), the test statistic $T(\theta)$ also has a similar quadratic form. Therefore, the null distribution of $T(\theta)$ can be asymptotically approximated by the same type of chi-squared distribution

$$\Pr\{T(\theta) > t(\theta) \mid H_0, \theta\} \approx \Pr\left\{ \chi_v^2 > v + \sqrt{2v} \left(\frac{t(\theta) - E(T(\theta))}{\sqrt{\mathrm{Var}(T(\theta))}} \right) \right\} \tag{6.25}$$

where χ_v^2 denotes a random variable having a chi-squared distribution with degrees of freedom v, where θ is omitted in the equations below,

$$E(T) = \sum_{i=1}^{n} \sum_{j=1}^{n} E(\delta_i \delta_j) a_{ij}$$

$$= p_1 \left(\sum_{i=1}^{n} \sum_{j=1}^{n} a_{ij} \right) = p_1 S_0 = \mu, \tag{6.26}$$

$$\mathrm{Var}(T) = (p_3 - p_1^2) S_0 + 2(p_1 - 4p_2 + 3p_3) \sum_{i=1}^{n} \sum_{j=1}^{n} a_{ij}^2$$

$$+ 4(p_2 - p_3) \sum_{i=1}^{n} \sum_{j=1}^{n} a_{ij} a_{i\cdot} = \sigma^2 \tag{6.27}$$

$$v = \frac{8}{(\sqrt{\beta_1(T)})^2} \tag{6.28}$$

$$\sqrt{\beta_1(T)} = \frac{E\{(T-\mu)^3\}}{\mathrm{Var}(T)^{1.5}} \quad \text{(skewness)} \tag{6.29}$$

$$E\{(T-\mu)^3\} = \sum_{r=1}^{5} p_r W_r - 3\mu\sigma^2 - \mu^3 \tag{6.30}$$

$$W_1 = 4\sum_{i=1}^{n}\sum_{j=1}^{n} a_{ij}^3$$

$$W_2 = \sum_{i=1}^{n}\sum_{j=1}^{n} \left\{ 24a_{ij}^2 a_{i\cdot} - 24a_{ij}^3 + 8a_{ij}\sum_{m=1}^{n} a_{im}a_{jm} \right\}$$

$$W_3 = \sum_{i=1}^{n}\sum_{j=1}^{n} \{6S_0 a_{ij}^2 + 52a_{ij}^3 - 96a_{ij}^2 a_{i\cdot} + 8a_{ij}a_{i\cdot}^2$$

$$+24a_{ij}a_{i\cdot}a_{j\cdot} - 24a_{ij}\sum_{m=1}^{n} a_{im}a_{jm} \bigg\}$$

$$W_4 = 12\sum_{i=1}^{n}\sum_{j=1}^{n} \{ -S_0 a_{ij}^2 - 4a_{ij}^3 + 10a_{ij}^2 a_{i\cdot} - a_{ij}a_{i\cdot}^2$$

$$-4a_{ij}a_{i\cdot}a_{j\cdot} + a_{i\cdot}^2 a_{j\cdot} + 2a_{ij}\sum_{m=1}^{n} a_{im}a_{jm} \bigg\}$$

$$W_5 = S_0^3 - W_1 - W_2 - W_3 - W_4$$

$$a_{i\cdot} = \sum_{j=1}^{n} a_{ij}$$

$$p_j = \prod_{l=0}^{j} \frac{n_0 - l}{n - l}$$

This type of approximation has already been shown to be a fairly good approximation for small sample sizes (Tango, 1990, 1995).

Null distribution of $P_{\min}$

The test statistic $P_{\min}$ is written as

$$P_{\min} \approx \min_{\theta_L \le \theta \le \theta_U} \mathrm{Pr}\left\{ \chi_v^2 > v + \sqrt{2v}\left(\frac{t(\theta) - E(T(\theta))}{\sqrt{\mathrm{Var}(T(\theta))}} \right) \right\}$$

$$= \mathrm{Pr}\left\{ \chi_v^2 > v + \sqrt{2v}\left(\frac{t(\theta^*) - E(T(\theta^*))}{\sqrt{\mathrm{Var}(T(\theta^*))}} \right) \right\} \tag{6.31}$$

Practical implementation of this procedure uses "line search" by discretization of θ. Regarding the selection of the lower bound θ_L, we would like to recommend θ_L such that $T(\theta_L) \geq 3$ since even the chi-square approximation is not so good for $T(\theta) \leq 3$ in general. A rational way of determining the upper bound θ_U without knowing the cluster size, on the other hand, would be to use an appropriate value for the lower tail of the distribution of distances between data points, say around 5% or 10%, because the percentage of the number of clustered cases can usually be assumed to be very small.

Monte Carlo hypothesis testing is required under the random labeling hypothesis to obtain the null distribution of $P_{\min}$ and the Monte Carlo simulated p-value (2.17).

Identification of local clustering areas

If the null hypothesis is rejected, then we would like to find the areas where clustering occurs. To search for such areas or cases, the statistic

$$C(j \mid \theta^*) = \sum_{i=1}^{n} \delta_i a_{ij}(\theta^*), \quad \text{for case } j \tag{6.32}$$

or

$$Q(j \mid \theta^*) = C(j \mid \theta^*)/T(\theta^*), \quad \text{for case } j \tag{6.33}$$

can be used, which denote the percentage of the jth case's contribution to the test statistic $T(\theta^*)$. Empirically, the cases with large $C(j \mid \theta^*)$ or $Q(j \mid \theta^*)$ are the cause of significant clustering.

6.4.3 Diggle and Chetwynd's Test

Note that this procedure is for comparing the degree of spatial clustering of cases with that of controls and is not for testing the null hypothesis of no clustering in the usual way.

Goal: To calculate the difference between the K-function for cases and that for controls and evaluate the significance of the difference. A significantly positive value would indicate *evidence of spatial clustering of cases that is larger than that of controls and would not always indicate evidence of spatial clustering of cases after being adjusted for heterogeneity of the spatial pattern of controls.* (For details, see Section 6.3.)
Null hypothesis H_0: (6.4)
Alternative hypothesis H_1: not H_0

Test statistic

Before applying this test, the study region A covering n data points must be defined and the area of the study region, $|A|$, must be calculated. Although I have already explained in Section 2.2 that there is no need for edge correction when testing the null hypothesis of no clustering, Diggle and Chetwynd's original procedure with the edge correction is described here in honor of the authors. Diggle and Chetwynd's test statistic is a combination of the information from a predefined discrete set of equally spaced distances s_k, $k = 1, ..., m$,

$$D = \sum_{k=1}^{m} \hat{D}(s_k) / \sqrt{\text{Var}\{\hat{D}(s_k)\}} \tag{6.34}$$

where $D(s)$ is the difference between the K-function (2.2) for cases and that for controls,

$$D(s) = K_{\text{case}}(s) - K_{\text{control}}(s) \tag{6.35}$$

Positive values of $D(s)$ suggest spatial aggregation of cases over and above the degree of spatial aggregation of controls. Estimates of K-functions using the notation in this chapter are given by

$$\hat{K}_{\text{case}}(s) = \frac{|A|}{n_0(n_0-1)} \sum_{i=1}^{n} \sum_{j=1}^{n} \delta_i \delta_j w_{ij} I(d_{ij} \leq s) \tag{6.36}$$

$$\hat{K}_{\text{control}}(s) = \frac{|A|}{n_1(n_1-1)} \sum_{i=1}^{n} \sum_{j=1}^{n} (1-\delta_i)(1-\delta_j) w_{ij} I(d_{ij} \leq s) \tag{6.37}$$

where w_{ij} ($w_{ii} = 0$) denote the reciprocal of the proportion of the circumference of the circle with center z_i and radius d_{ij} that lies within A and $I(\cdot)$ is the indicator function. Furthermore, for any integer m and $r \geq 1$, by writing $m^{(r)} = m(m-1)\cdots(m-r+1)$, we have

$$\text{Cov}\{\hat{D}(s), \hat{D}(u)\} = |A|^2 (n_0^{(2)} n_1^{(2)})^{-2} \left\{ (n_1^{(2)})^2 \mu_1 - 2(n_0^{(2)} n_1^{(2)}) \mu_2 + (n_0^{(2)})^2 \mu_3 \right\} \tag{6.38}$$

where

$$\mu_1 = (n_0^{(4)}/n^{(4)})(WV - 4Z + 2X) + 4((n_0^{(3)}/n^{(3)}))(Z - X) + 2(n_0^{(2)}/n^{(2)})X$$

$$\mu_2 = (n_0^{(2)} n_1^{(2)}/n^{(4)})(WV - 4Z + 2X)$$

$$\mu_3 = (n_1^{(4)}/n^{(4)})(WV - 4Z + 2X) + 4((n_1^{(3)}/n^{(3)}))(Z - X) + 2(n_1^{(2)}/n^{(2)})X$$

$$W = \sum_{i=1}^{n} \sum_{j=1}^{n} (w_{ij} + w_{ji}) I(d_{ij} \leq s)/2$$

$$V = \sum_{i=1}^{n} \sum_{j=1}^{n} (w_{ij} + w_{ji}) I(d_{ij} \leq u)/2$$

$$X = \sum_{i=1}^{n} \sum_{j=1}^{n} (w_{ij} + w_{ji})^2 I(d_{ij} \leq s) I(d_{ij} \leq u)/4$$

$$Z = \sum_{i=1}^{n} \left\{ \sum_{j=1}^{n} (w_{ij} + w_{ji}) I(d_{ij} \leq s)/2 \right\} \left\{ \sum_{k=1}^{n} (w_{ik} + w_{ki}) I(d_{ik} \leq u)/2 \right\}$$

However, it seems to me that the Max test

$$D = D_{\max} = \max_{k=1,\dots,m} \hat{D}(s_k)/\sqrt{\text{Var}\{\hat{D}(s_k)\}} \tag{6.39}$$

which was Diggle and Chetwynd's third candidate for a possible test statistic, would be more powerful than the SUM test (6.34) for detecting disease clustering.

Null distribution

The approximate distribution of the test statistic (6.34) under the null hypothesis could be normal,

$$Z = \frac{D}{\sqrt{\text{Var}(D)}} \sim N(0,1) \tag{6.40}$$

where

$$E(D) = 0, \quad \text{Var}(D) = m + 2 \sum_{j=1}^{m} \sum_{k=1}^{j-1} \text{Corr}\{\hat{D}(s_j), \hat{D}(s_k)\}$$

However, Monte Carlo hypothesis testing is required under the random labeling hypothesis to obtain a more accurate null distribution of Z_k and the Monte Carlo simulated p-value (2.17).

Pointwise tolerance limits

A plot of the estimated test statistic $\hat{D}(s_k)$ evaluated at a discrete set of equally spaced values s_k, $k = 1,\dots,m$, together with approximate 95% pointwise tolerance limits $\pm 2\sqrt{\text{Var}\{\hat{D}(s_k)\}}$ evaluated from (6.38) are helpful in the interpretation of the test results.

Software

To apply Diggle and Chetwynd's method, we can use the package **splancs** (Spatial and Space-Time Point Pattern Analysis) (Rowlingson and Diggle, 1993) which can easily be installed in the R system. The original sources can be accessed at

http://www.maths.lancs.ac.uk/~rowlings/Splancs/

6.4.4 Kulldorff's Spatial Scan Statistic

Goal: To detect the most likely *circular* hot-spot cluster and secondary clusters, if any, within the study area and evaluate its (their) statistical significance. The finding that the most likely cluster is significant would suggest evidence for the existence of a localized cluster within the study area.

Null hypothesis and alternative hypothesis

$$
\begin{aligned}
H_0 &: \text{ disease risk is constant over the area, expressed in (6.5)} \\
H_1 &: \text{ there is an elevated risk within the window } \mathbf{Z} \qquad (6.41) \\
& \text{ as compared with outside it}
\end{aligned}
$$

where $\mathbf{Z}$ denotes a *circular window* centered at some point z.

Test statistic (under the Bernoulli model)

$$
\lambda = \sup_{\mathbf{Z} \in \mathscr{Z}} \left(\frac{n_0(\mathbf{Z})}{n(\mathbf{Z})} \right)^{n_0(\mathbf{Z})} \left(\frac{n(\mathbf{Z}) - n_0(\mathbf{Z})}{n(\mathbf{Z})} \right)^{n(\mathbf{Z}) - n_0(\mathbf{Z})} \left(\frac{n_0 - n_0(\mathbf{Z})}{n - n(\mathbf{Z})} \right)^{n_0 - n_0(\mathbf{Z})}
$$
$$
\left(\frac{[n - n(\mathbf{Z})] - [n_0 - n_0(\mathbf{Z})]}{n - n(\mathbf{Z})} \right)^{[n - n(\mathbf{Z})] - [n_0 - n_0(\mathbf{Z})]} I\left(\frac{n_0(\mathbf{Z})}{n(\mathbf{Z})} > \frac{n_0 - n_0(\mathbf{Z})}{n - n(\mathbf{Z})} \right)
$$
$$
(6.42)
$$

where $n_0(\mathbf{Z})$ and $n(\mathbf{Z})$ denote the observed number of cases and the observed number of cases and controls within the window $\mathbf{Z}$, respectively, and window $\mathbf{Z}$ to be scanned by the spatial scan statistic is included in the set

$$
\mathscr{Z} = \{ \mathbf{Z}_{ik} \mid 1 \leq i \leq m, \ 1 \leq k \leq K_i \}
$$

where $\mathbf{Z}_{ik}$, $k = 1, \ldots, K_i$, denotes the window composed by the $(k - 1)$ nearest neighbors to case z_i. The value of K_i depends on the starting region i so that the radius of the circle varies from zero upward until 50% of the total points n are covered. The window $\mathbf{Z}^*$ that attains the maximum likelihood is defined as the *most* *likely cluster* (MLC). If the most likely cluster is significant, then we can search for significant *secondary clusters* that do not overlap with the most likely cluster, if any, and order them according to their likelihood ratio test statistic.

Null distribution

Monte Carlo hypothesis testing is required under the random labeling hypothesis to obtain the null distribution of P_{min} and the Monte Carlo simulated p-value (2.17). The p-value of a secondary cluster is obtained by comparing its likelihood with the null distribution of λ.

Software

SaTScan: http://www.satscan.org/

6.5 Illustration with Real Data

In these illustrations, the Monte Carlo test consists of $N_{rep} = 9,999$ or 999 replications of randomly labeled data generated under the null hypothesis, depending on the situation.

6.5.1 Leukemia and lymphoma in North Humberside

Cuzick and Edwards (1990) analyzed 62 cases of childhood leukemia and lymphoma diagnosed in North Humberside between 1974 and 1986 and 141 controls selected at random from entries in the birth register for January 7 or June 7 for each of the years 1974–1986. Centroids of postal codes of home addresses were used to obtain grid references for mapping and these data, which were listed in their Table 6, are shown in Figure 6.1, in which the unit of measurement is 100 m.

k nearest neighbors model

First, let us apply Cuzick and Edwards' k nearest neighbors test or Tango's test with k nearest neighbors model. The values of $T(k)$, their means, variances, and skewness under the null hypothesis and p-value based upon approximate $N(0,1)$, p-values based upon chi-squared and simulated p-values are given in Table 6.1(a) for $k = 1, ..., 10$, which are reproduced from Tango (2007).

These results are derived using the tie evaluation approach described in Cuzick and Edwards (1990), as there were several ties in the data. Surprisingly, variances and p-values based upon $N(0,1)$ do not coincide with those of Cuzick and Edwards' results shown in their Table 5 but completely coincide with those of Jacquez's re-

Table 6.1 Analysis of leukemia and lymphoma data in the North Humberside area from Tango (2007).

No.	θ	Observed value $t(\theta)$	$E(T(\theta))$	$\mathrm{Var}(T(\theta))$	Skewness	$N(0,1)$	χ^2_ν	Monte Carlo
(a) the $k(=\theta)$ nearest neighbors model								
1	1	24.500	18.723	16.980	.104	.0805	.0828	.0900
2	2	52.500	37.446	34.574	.171	.0052	.0077	.0086
3	3	76.500	56.168	53.355	.212	.0027	.0049*	.0063
4	4	95.833	74.891	72.787	.248	.0071	.0112	.0124
5	5	115.167	93.614	92.139	.284	.0124	.0183	.0188
6	6	128.000	112.337	111.911	.311	.0694	.0762	.0774
7	7	143.500	131.059	131.970	.337	.1394	.1403	.1399
8	8	160.000	149.782	154.360	.353	.2054	.1994	.1962
9	9	177.000	168.505	177.488	.370	.2619	.2498	.2496
10	10	194.000	187.228	202.956	.383	.3173	.2998	.3013

$P_{\min} = 0.00490$ ($k^*=3$), adjusted p-value $= 223/10000 = 0.0223$

No.	θ	Observed value $t(\theta)$	$E(T(\theta))$	$\mathrm{Var}(T(\theta))$	Skewness	$N(0,1)$	χ^2_ν	Monte Carlo
(b) the double exponential clinal model								
1	300 (m)	6.378	5.108	5.870	.504	.3000	.2789	.2817
2	400	10.969	7.590	8.621	.458	.1249	.1276	.1266
3	500	15.878	10.451	12.051	.443	.0590	.0688	.0670
4	600	20.767	13.590	15.959	.431	.0362	.0468	.0469
5	700	25.664	16.984	20.584	.419	.0279	.0382	.0385
6	800	30.511	20.718	26.114	.412	.0276	.0378*	.0392
7	900	35.409	24.853	32.692	.411	.0324	.0427	.0421
8	1000	40.396	29.329	40.672	.414	.0413	.0516	.0504
9	1100	45.586	34.136	49.907	.419	.0525	.0624	.0643
10	1200	51.134	39.227	60.666	.424	.0632	.0724	.0751
11	1300	56.754	44.703	73.193	.428	.0795	.0873	.0892
12	1400	62.615	50.385	87.430	.431	.0955	.1016	.1008
13	1500	68.541	56.360	103.429	.432	.1155	.1193	.1174

$P_{\min} = 0.0378$ ($\theta^*=800$), adjusted p-value $= 853/10000 = 0.0853$

sults (1994) shown in his Table 1. According to personal communication with Dr. Jacquez via email, it also seems that he could not replicate Cuzick and Edwards' published result for variance. Therefore, it seems to me that there is a problem with Cuzick and Edwards' results. Furthermore, Cuzick and Edwards gave simulated significance levels based upon 1000 simulations and showed that asymptotically estimated significance levels agree well with the simulated significance levels. However, our results show that there is a small but nonnegligible amount of skewness irrespective of the value of k, indicating that the normal approximation is poor. Thus we can see in greater detail that (1) normal approximated p-values are nonnegligibly smaller than those simulated for $k = 1,...,6$ and (2), conversely, are larger than those simulated for $k > 7$. On the other hand, chi-square approximated p-values are shown to agree better with simulated p-values (Figure 6.3). Table 6.1(a) shows that a value of $k^* = 3$, corresponding to a cluster of size 4, appears to give the most sig-

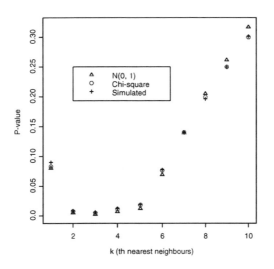

Fig. 6.3 Comparison of normal approximated p-values, chi-square approximated p-values, and simulated p-values for the k nearest neighbors model.

nificance results, $p = 0.0049$. This p-value is the 223rd largest among 9999 $P_{\min}$'s. Therefore, the adjusted p-value of $P_{\min}$ is $223/(9999+1) = 0.0223$, which leads to a statistically significant clustering of cases at a conventional significance level of 0.05.

To see the clustering areas, we considered the statistic of each case's contribution $C(j \mid \theta^*)$, whose frequency distribution is shown in Figure 6.4, and identified 18 cases with $C(j \mid k^* = 3) \geq 2$, which are indicated by a "circle" in Figure 6.5. From this figure, we may observe that the k nearest neighbors test result suggests a pattern of clustering at small *nearest neighbors*; i.e., between cases falling within the three nearest neighbors of cases. However, we cannot conclude that we have observed a pattern of significant clustering at small *distances* since (1) the median and 75th percentile of distances among the cases with $C(j \mid k^* = 3) \geq 2$ and their three nearest neighbors that are cases are 447 m and 712 m, and (2) we can observe seven cases $\{1, 4, 7, 10, 26, 36, 46\}$ in which their distance to the corresponding three nearest neighbors is larger than 3 km (large distance), except for the distance between 1 and 26 ($d_{1,26} = 707$ m), and that their contributions to the significant test result are large or at least not negligible.

A part of the result shown in Table 6.1(a) can be reproduced by using the R function **TangoCNN.index** (Appendix) shown below. The input data required for this program have two different files:

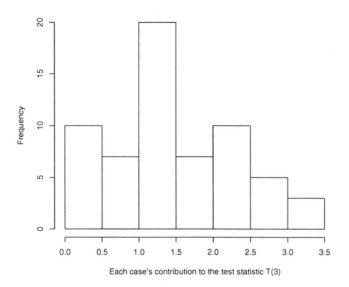

Fig. 6.4 Distribution of $C(j \mid k^* = 3)$.

1. Case file ("case" in the R program):
   Format: $<$ case ID $>$ $<$ y-coordinate $>$ $<$ x-coordinate $>$
2. Coordinate file ("cont" in the R program):
   Format: $<$ case ID $>$ $<$ y-coordinate $>$ $<$ x-coordinate $>$

Furthermore, we need a sequence of values of cluster size θ ("k" in the R program) and we considered ten values $(1, 2, ..., 10)$.

Output from the R function TangoCNN.index

```
> k< − 1:10; Nrep< − 999
> case< − scan("LKcase.geo",list(id=0, x=0, y=0))
> cont< − scan("LKcont.geo",list(id=0, x=0, y=0))
> out< − TangoCNN.index(case, cont, k, Nrep)
> signif(out$Pmin,4)
[1] 0.083 0.008 0.005 0.011 0.018 0.076 0.140 0.199 0.249 0.299
> out$k.min
[1] 3
> out$p.value
[1] 0.033
```

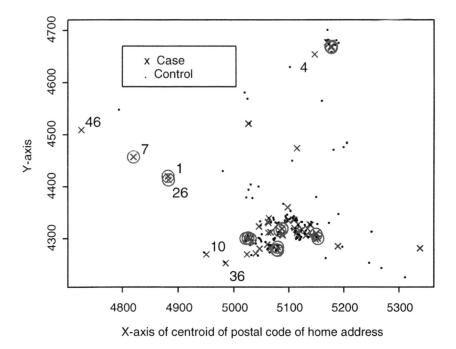

Fig. 6.5 Locations of 62 cases of childhood leukemia and lymphoma and 141 controls between 1974 and 1986 in the North Humberside area and the results of the k nearest neighbors model applied to these data. The circle represents the case j, whose contribution to the test statistic with $k^* = 3$ is large, i.e., $C(j \mid k^* = 3) \geq 2$. The cases with numbers shown indicate that the distance to the nearest neighbors is larger than 3 km except for case 1 and case 26 (distance 707 m); their contribution to the test statistic is not negligible.

In this example, we consider the test statistic

$$P_{\min} = \min_{k \in \{1, \ldots, 10\}} \Pr\{T(k) > t(k) \mid H_0, k\}$$

and obtain $P_{\min} = 0.0049$ at $k^* = 3$. The adjusted p-value of $P_{\min}$ was $33/(999 + 1) = 0.033$ using Monte Carlo testing with 999 replicates.

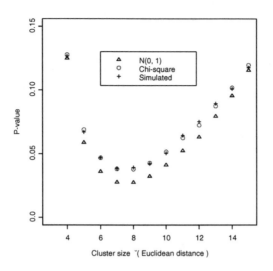

Fig. 6.6 Comparison of normal approximated p-values, chi-square approximated p-values, and simulated p-values for the double exponential clinal model.

The double exponential clinal model

Next, we shall apply the double exponential clinal model (6.22). The maximum, median, and minimum distances between data points are 65.2 km, 8.96 km and 0.0 km, respectively. As the fifth percentile of the distribution of distance between data points is about 1.5 km, we shall take a sequence of values of θ as 300, 400, ..., 1500 m to obtain the test statistic $P_{\min}$

$$P_{\min} = \min_{\theta \in \{300,\ 400,...,1500\}} \Pr\{T(\theta) > t(\theta) \mid H_0, \theta\} \tag{6.43}$$

where $\theta_L = 300$ is taken since it is the minimum integer such that $T(\theta_L) \geq 300$. Table 6.1(b) summarizes our results in the same way as Table 6.1(a). Here also we can see that the normal approximated p-values are liberal and the chi-square approximation is good compared with simulated p-values (Figure 6.6). Table 6.1(b) shows that a value of cluster size $\theta^* = 800$ appears to give the most significant results, $p = 0.0378$. However, this p-value is the 853rd largest among 9999 $P_{\min}$'s. Therefore, the adjusted p-value of $P_{\min}$ is 0.0853, indicating that there is no significant clustering of cases under the exponential clinal model. Although the test result is nonsignificant, let us examine the cases contributing to the nonadjusted $T(800)$. To see this, we examined the distribution of $Q(j \mid \theta^*)$ (Figure 6.7) and chose 17 cases that satisfied the condition $Q(j \mid \theta^* = 800) \geq 2.5\%$ and have identified them by "circle" in Figure 6.8. It can be seen that these areas detected by the clinal model are quite similar to those indicated by the three nearest neighbors model except for

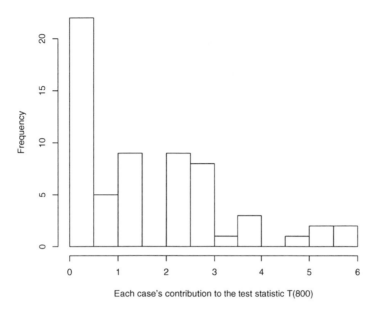

Fig. 6.7 Distribution of $Q(j \mid \theta^* = 800)$.

the seven outlying cases stated above that were not indicated in the clinal model. This is easily understood since most of the distances from these outlying cases to their three nearest neighbors are far larger than the cluster size $\theta^* = 800$.

These results may be summarized as follows: (1) As the k nearest neighbors model gives equal weight to all the nearest neighbors of each case, we may say that these seven cases situated far apart from each other made a large contribution to the test statistic and caused an *apparent* statistically significant clustering and (2) if we believe the model of decline in risk with distance, the significant clustering according to the nearest neighbors test cannot be accepted. However, as we do not know the truth, detailed medical investigation of these seven cases and their neighbors would be quite important.

A part of the result shown in Table 6.1(b) can also be reproduced by using the R function **TangoCDE.index** (Appendix) shown below. The input data required for this program are the same as for the **TangoCNN.index**. In this case, we need a sequence of values of cluster size θ ("s" in the R program) $(300, 400, ..., 1500)$.

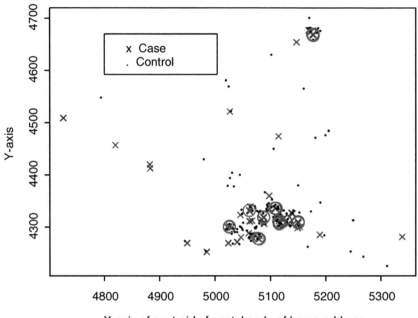

Fig. 6.8 Results of the exponential clinal model applied to data on the locations of 62 cases of childhood leukemia and lymphoma and 141 controls. The circle represents the case j, whose contribution to the test statistic with $\theta^* = 800$ is large; i.e., $Q(j \mid \theta^* = 800) \geq 2.5\%$.

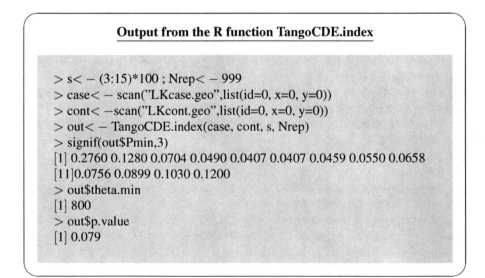

Output from the R function TangoCDE.index

```
> s< − (3:15)*100 ; Nrep< − 999
> case< − scan("LKcase.geo",list(id=0, x=0, y=0))
> cont< −scan("LKcont.geo",list(id=0, x=0, y=0))
> out< − TangoCDE.index(case, cont, s, Nrep)
> signif(out$Pmin,3)
[1] 0.2760 0.1280 0.0704 0.0490 0.0407 0.0407 0.0459 0.0550 0.0658
[11]0.0756 0.0899 0.1030 0.1200
> out$theta.min
[1] 800
> out$p.value
[1] 0.079
```

In this example, we consider the test statistic

$$P_{\min} = \min_{k \in \{300,\ldots,1500\}} \Pr\{T(\theta) > t(\theta) \mid H_0, \theta\}$$

and obtain $P_{\min} = 0.04069$ at $\theta^* = 800$. The adjusted p-value of $P_{\min}$ was $79/(999 + 1) = 0.079$ using Monte Carlo testing with 999 replicates.

Diggle and Chetwynd's test To compare the degree of spatial clustering of cases with that of controls, we shall apply the Diggle and Chetwynd method using the package **splancs**. As the study region $|A|$ covering all the data points, we used the same convex polygonal study region as Diggle and Chetwynd used, which approximates the administrative boundary of North Humberside. To do this, we use the R program

---

R program for Figure 6.9

```
cases< − spoints(scan("LKcase.txt"))
conts< − spoints(scan("LKcont.txt"))
polys< − spoints(scan("LKpoly.txt"))
pointmap(cases,xlim=c(4600,5400), ylim=c(4100,4800),pch=4,
xlab="X-axis of centroid of postal code of home address",ylab="Y-
axis")
legend(4700,4800,c(" x Case"," . Control"))
pointmap(conts, add=T, pch=".")
polymap(polys,add=T)
```

---

where the three files LKcase.txt, LKcont.txt, and LKpoly.txt denote the x and y coordinates for cases, controls, and the vertices of a polygon, respectively. The result is shown in Figure 6.9.

R program for Figure 6.10

```
s< − seq(from=1, to=10, len=10)
Kcase< − khat(cases, polys, s)
Kcont< − khat(conts, polys, s)
SEcc < − secal(cases, conts, polys, s)
matplot(s, 2*cbind(SEcc, −SEcc), type='l', lty=3, col=1)
lines(s, Kcase−Kcont, lwd=2)
> signif((Kcase−Kcont)/SEcc,3)
[1] 0.343 0.556 1.730 1.020 2.180 1.980 1.420 0.755 0.466 0.209
```

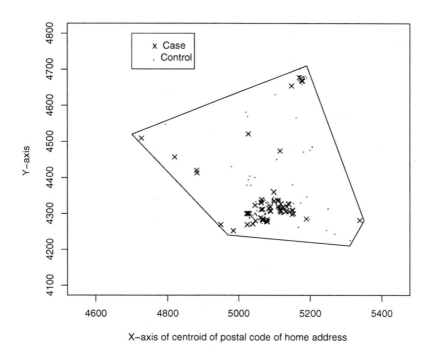

Fig. 6.9 Locations of 62 cases of childhood leukemia and lymphoma and 141 controls between 1974 and 1986 in the North Humberside area and the convex polygonal study region $|A|$ that approximates the administrative boundary of the area, that was used in the analysis.

Then, we made a plot of the estimated test statistic $\hat{D}(s_k)$ evaluated at a discrete set of equally spaced values $s_k = k$, $k = 1,...,10$ (unit: 100 m) together with approximate 95% pointwise tolerance limits $\pm 2\sqrt{\text{Var}\{\hat{D}(s_k)\}}$ evaluated from (6.38), which are shown in Figure 6.10. The estimated $\hat{D}(s_k)$ strayed just beyond the upper tolerance limit at $s = 5$ (500 m), i.e., its standardized value was 2.18 at $s = 5$, which could suggest weak evidence of spatial clustering of cases that is larger than that of controls within 500 m. These analyses were carried out using the R programs above.

Output from the R function DiggleChetwynd.test

```
> sum((Kcase–Kcont)/SEcc)
[1] 10.64963
> max((Kcase–Kcont)/SEcc)
[1] 2.176142
>Nrep< – 999
>s< – seq(from=1, to=10, len=10)
>out< – DiggleChetwynd.test(cases,conts,polys,s,Nrep)
>out$Sum.p.value
[1] 0.102
>out$Max.p.value
[1] 0.093
```

As the next analysis, we performed two Monte Carlo tests with $N_{rep} = 999$ based on the Sum test statistic D and the Max test statistic D_{max} using the R function **DiggleChetwynd.test** (Appendix). The observed Sum test statistic was $D = 10.65$ and the Max test statistic was $D_{max} = 2.18$ at $s = 500$ m. The simulated p-value of the observed $D = 10.65$ was $p = 0.102$ and that of the observed $D_{max} = 2.18$ was 0.093, which also suggests weak evidence of spatial clustering of cases that is larger than that of controls within 500 m.

6.5.2 Early Medieval Grave Sites

We shall apply our proposed methods to data on 143 early medieval grave sites described in Waller and Gotway (2004) that originally appeared in Alt and Vach (1991). The anthropologists and archaeologists conducted an investigation of an early medieval burial ground in Neresheim, Germany, to examine whether the particular culture tended to place grave sites according to family unit. They used inherited features in the teeth of excavated skeletons to mark a subset of sites. Table 5.2 of Waller and Gotway's book includes 30 grave sites where skeletons have affected teeth (graves of "affected individuals") and 113 where they did not. The research question here is whether there is any clustering of affected sites. Figure 6.2 shows the locations of affected and nonaffected sites.

k **nearest neighbors model**

First, we apply the *k* nearest neighbors model. Table 6.2(a) summarizes the results for $k = 1, ..., 10$. Here also, it is shown that while the approximated p-values based upon the normal distribution are liberal, the chi-square approximated p-values are

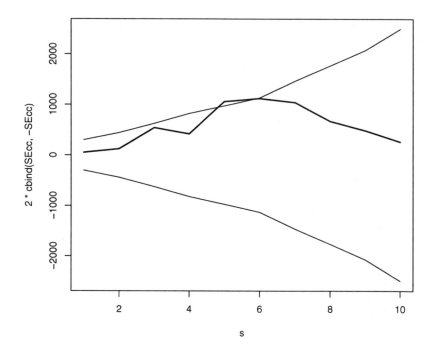

Fig. 6.10 Estimated test statistic $\hat{D}(s_k)$ evaluated at a discrete set of equally spaced values $s_k = k$, $k = 1,...,10$ (unit: 100 m) together with approximate 95% pointwise tolerance limits $\pm 2\sqrt{\text{Var}\{\hat{D}(s_k)\}}$ (dotted line) for data on 62 cases of childhood leukemia and lymphoma and 141 controls between 1974 and 1986 in the North Humberside area.

close to the simulated p-values. A value of $k = 3$ appears to give the most significant results, $T(k) = 32$ and $p = 0.0042$. This p-value is the 167th largest among 9999 $P_{\min}$'s. Therefore, the adjusted p-value of $P_{\min}$ is 0.0167 and, as a consequence, we may conclude that there could be a statistically significant clustering of cases, especially between affected grave sites *falling within three nearest neighbors of affected grave sites*. In Figure 6.11, the 14 cases

$$\{11, 30, 39, 42, 62, 67, 78, 80, 90, 98, 118, 131, 132, 142\}$$

are indicated by circles, whose contribution to the test statistic is large; i.e., $C(j \mid k^* = 3) = 1.5, 2.0$, and 3.0.

Table 6.2 Analysis of a data set of early medieval grave site locations consisting of affected and nonaffected grave sites.

No.	θ	Observed value $t(\theta)$	$E(T(\theta))$	$Var(T(\theta))$	Skewness	$N(0,1)$	χ_v^2	Monte Carlo
							p-value	
(a) the $k(=\theta)$ nearest neighbors model								
1	1	10.000	6.127	6.894	.301	.0701	.0767	.1014
2	2	20.000	12.254	14.337	.274	.0204	.0271	.0364
3	3	32.000	18.380	21.697	.294	.0017	.0042*	.0055
4	4	40.000	24.507	29.235	.342	.0021	.0054	.0069
5	5	45.000	30.634	36.936	.356	.0090	.0157	.0191
6	6	51.000	36.761	44.486	.397	.0164	.0253	.0280
7	7	58.000	42.887	52.406	.424	.0184	.0281	.0305
8	8	64.000	49.014	60.119	.447	.0266	.0375	.0386
9	9	73.000	55.141	67.900	.468	.0151	.0252	.0252
10	10	80.000	61.268	75.680	.494	.0156	.0263	.0262

$P_{\min} = 0.00425$ ($k^*=3$), adjusted *p*-value $= 167/10000 = 0.0167$

(b)the double exponential clinal model								
1	25.000	3.241	.139	.225	3.399	3×10^{-11}	.0020	.0017
2	50.000	3.776	.187	.297	3.094	2×10^{-11}	.0016*	.0017
3	75.000	3.897	.252	.368	2.603	9×10^{-10}	.0017	.0017
4	100.000	3.942	.330	.466	2.256	6×10^{-8}	.0024	.0023
5	125.000	3.962	.427	.574	2.058	2×10^{-6}	.0036	.0031
6	150.000	3.974	.552	.697	1.892	2×10^{-5}	.0057	.0043
7	175.000	3.981	.698	.842	1.725	.0002	.0088	.0080
8	200.000	3.985	.862	1.009	1.564	.0009	.0135	.0169
9	225.000	3.988	1.044	1.197	1.423	.0036	.0206	.0234
10	250.000	3.991	1.251	1.404	1.300	.0104	.0311	.0329
11	275.000	3.992	1.473	1.627	1.198	.0242	.0461	.0483
12	300.000	4.165	1.733	1.860	1.111	.0373	.0577	.0607
13	325.000	4.350	2.024	2.109	1.037	.0546	.0720	.0762
14	350.000	4.668	2.349	2.374	.971	.0662	.0811	.0858
15	375.000	5.133	2.718	2.657	.913	.0692	.0832	.0883
16	400.000	5.627	3.111	2.970	.861	.0722	.0852	.0905
17	425.000	6.274	3.566	3.306	.815	.0682	.0816	.0876
18	450.000	6.916	4.040	3.673	.776	.0667	.0800	.0854
19	475.000	7.607	4.565	4.081	.741	.0660	.0791	.0848
20	500.000	8.462	5.130	4.530	.711	.0587	.0724	.0779

$P_{\min} = 0.0016$ ($\theta^*=50$), adjusted *p*-value $= 49/10000 = 0.0049$

The double exponential clinal model

We shall next apply the exponential clinal model (6.22). As the fifth percentile of distribution of distance between data points is 670, we shall take a sequence of values of θ as 25, 50, 75,..., 475, 500 to obtain the test statistic $P_{\min}$

$$P_{\min} = \min_{\theta \in \{25,50,75,\ldots,500\}} \Pr\{T(\theta) > t(\theta) \mid H_0, \theta\}$$

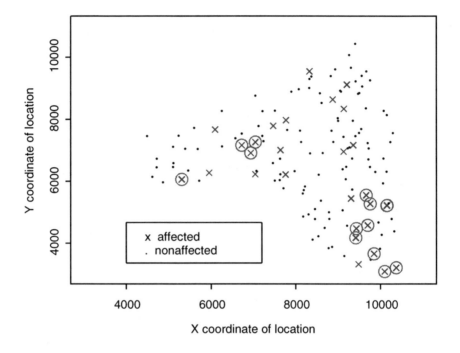

Fig. 6.11 Locations of 143 early medieval grave sites and the results of the k nearest neighbors model applied to these data. The circle represents the 14 cases $\{11, 30, 39, 42, 62, 67, 78, 80, 90, 98, 118, 131, 132, 142\}$ whose contribution to the test statistic with $k^* = 3$ is large, i.e., $C(j \mid k^* = 3) = 1.5, 2.0$, and 3.0.

where $\theta_L = 25$ is taken since it satisfies $T(\theta_L) \geq 3$. Table 6.2(b) summarizes the results, where we can easily see that there is a substantial amount of skewness for the test statistic $T(\theta)$ and the resultant approximated p-values based upon $N(0, 1)$ are quite liberal for all the values of θ considered here. The chi-square approximation, however, coincides well with the simulated p-values. Table 6.2(b) shows that a value of cluster size $\theta = 50$ appears to give the most significant results, $T(50) = 3.776$ and $p = 0.0016$. This p-value is the 49th largest among 9999 P_{min}'s. Therefore, the adjusted p-value of P_{min} is 0.0049, indicating that we could detect a significant clustering of cases by using the exponential clinal model. The four cases $\{20, 42, 80, 118\}$ indicated by circles in Figure 6.12 have the largest contri-

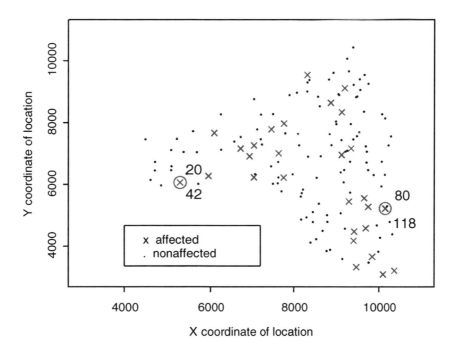

Fig. 6.12 Results of the exponential clinal model applied to data on the locations of 143 early medieval grave sites. The circle represents the four cases $\{20,42,80,118\}$ that have the largest contribution to the test statistic with $\theta^* = 50$ in the sense that the test statistic $T(50)$ is the sum of only these four cases' contributions $C(j \mid \theta^* = 50)$, $j = 20,40,80,118$. Cases 20 and 42 are situated at nearly the same location, $(5305,6065)$ and $(5306,6065)$, respectively. Cases 80 and 118 are also situated at nearly the same location, $(10156,5225)$ and $(10148,5222)$, respectively. Therefore, these two circles are seen as one in the figure.

bution to the test statistic in the sense that the test statistic $T(50)$ is the sum of only these four cases' contributions; namely, $C(20 \mid 3) = 0.998$, $C(42 \mid 3) = 0.998$, $C(80 \mid 3) = 0.890$, and $C(118 \mid 3) = 0.890$. The sum of these four values is equal to $T(50) = 3.776$. The reason is the following. Cases 20 and 42 are situated at nearly the same location, $(5305,6065)$ and $(5306,6065)$, respectively, and the distance between them is 1. Cases 80 and 118 are also situated at nearly the same location, $(10156,5225)$ and $(10148,5222)$, respectively, and the distance is 8.54. Therefore,

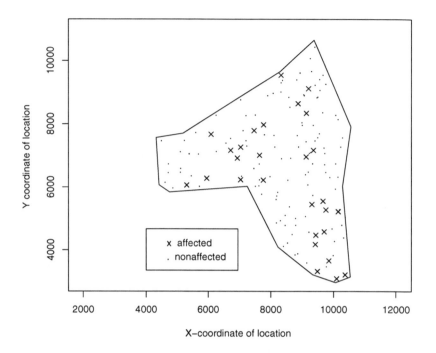

Fig. 6.13 Locations of 143 early medieval grave sites. The polygon surrounding the data points is used as the edge of the study region in the Diggle and Chetwynd method.

we conclude that the significant clustering detected by the clinal model is driven primarily by these two quite close pairs, which is a different interpretation from the significant clustering resulting from application of the three nearest neighbors model. The tendency of a dominant influence of these four cases was not altered for the wide range of values $\theta = 25 \sim 300$.

In this example, we omitted the application of the R functions **TangoCNN.index** and **TangoCDE.index** since the usage of these functions is the same as for childhood leukemia data.

Diggle and Chetwynd's test

To compare the degree of spatial clustering of cases with that of controls, we shall apply the Diggle and Chetwynd method using the package **splancs**. As the study region $| A |$ covering all the data points, we used the polygon shown in Figure 6.13, which was made using the **getpoly()** command of **splancs** and an R program similar to the previous example, where the two files GRcase.txt and GRcont.txt denote the x

and y coordinates for cases and controls, respectively. The result is shown in Figure 6.13.

R program for Figure 6.13

```
cases< −spoint(scan("GRcase.txt"))
conts< − spoint(scan("GRcont.txt"))
polys< − getpoly()
pointmap(cases,xlim=c(3000,11000), ylim=c(3000,11000),pch=4,
xlab="X-coordinate of location ", ylab="Y coordinate of location")
legend(4000,4670,c(" x affected"," . nonaffected"))
pointmap(conts, add=T, pch=".")
polymap(polys,add=T)
```

R program for Figure 6.14

```
s< − seq(from=25, to=500, len=20)
Kcase< − khat(cases, polys, s)
Kcont< − khat(conts, polys, s)
SEcc < − secal(cases, conts, polys, s)
matplot(s, 2*cbind(SEcc, −SEcc), type='l', lty=3, col=1)
lines(s, Kcase−Kcont, lwd=2)
> signif((Kcase−Kcont)/SEcc,3)
[1] 6.6300 3.8000 3.8000 2.2500 1.390 1.0300 0.7220 0.4330 0.0468
[10] −0.2640 −0.4490 1.7600 1.6100 1.9700 2.4400 2.3000 2.1800
1.8200
[20] 1.1700 1.6300
```

Then, we made a plot of the estimated test statistic $\hat{D}(s_k)$ evaluated at a discrete set of equally spaced values $s_k = 25k$, $k = 1,...,20$, together with approximate 95% pointwise tolerance limits $\pm 2\sqrt{\mathrm{Var}\{\hat{D}(s_k)\}}$ evaluated from (6.38), which are shown in Figure 6.14. The estimated $\hat{D}(s_k)$ strayed beyond the upper tolerance limit at $s < 100$ units, i.e., their standardized values were $6.63, 3.80, 3.80, 2.25$ at $s = 25, 50, 75, 100$ units, which could suggest evidence of spatial clustering of cases that is larger than that of controls within 100 units. These analyses were carried out using the R programs above.

Output from the R function DiggleChetwynd.test

```
> sum((Kcase–Kcont)/SEcc)
[1] 36.26721
> max((Kcase–Kcont)/SEcc)
[1] 6.631705
>Nrep< − 999
>s< − seq(from=25, to=500, len=20)
>out< − DiggleChetwynd.test(cases,conts,polys,s,Nrep)
>out$Sum.p.value
[1] 0.013
>out$Max.p.value
[1] 0.0015
```

As the next analysis, we performed two Monte Carlo tests with $N_{rep} = 999$ based on the Sum test statistic D and the Max test statistic D_{max} using the R function **DiggleChetwynd.test** (Appendix). The observed Sum test statistic was $D = 36.27$ and the Max test statistic was $D_{max} = 6.63$ at $s = 25$. The simulated p-value of the observed $D = 36.27$ was $p = 0.013$ and that of the observed $D_{max} = 6.63$ was 0.0015, which also suggests evidence of differences in the degree of spatial clustering between cases and controls within a distance of about 100 units.

6.6 Discussion

In this chapter, we have illustrated three procedures, Tango's clustering index based on (1) the k-nearest neighbors model and (2) double exponential clinal model and (3) Diggle and Chetwynd's K-function procedure, with two real data sets. Cuzick and Edwards' test statistic is included in Tango's clustering index with k nearest neighbors model, but Tango's test improves on theirs in terms of (i) providing a better asymptotic distribution, (ii) coping with the difficulty in choosing k, and (iii) providing a procedure for estimating the areas of clustering.

It should be noted again that Diggle and Chetwynd's test should be used when we are interested in comparing the degree of spatial clustering of cases with that of controls. In their method, the Max test (6.39) was illustrated to be more powerful than the Sum test (6.34) as expected using two real data sets.

Two kinds of real data illustrated here provided us with an interesting question: "Which is the appropriate metric, nearest neighbors or Euclidean distance?" If the scales of the spatial clustering are related to a Euclidean metric rather than a nearest neighbors metric, then the model based upon the former seems to be appropriate and vice versa. Therefore, expert rather than statistical evaluation of the relationship

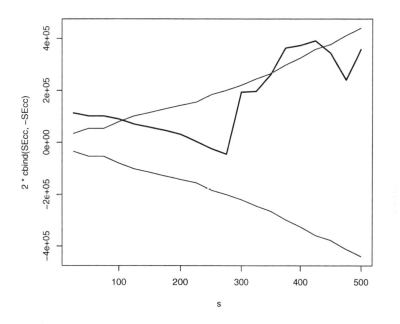

Fig. 6.14 Estimated test statistic $\hat{D}(s_k)$ evaluated at a discrete set of equally spaced approximate 95% pointwise tolerance limits $\pm 2\sqrt{\mathrm{Var}\{\hat{D}(s_k)\}}$ (dotted line) for data on the locations of 143 early medieval grave sites.

among cases, especially cases far apart that contributed to the test statistic, becomes very important to judge which is most appropriate.

When we are interested in detecting localized clusters and evaluating their significance, we should use Kulldorff's spatial scan statistic instead of the tests above.

Chapter 7
Tests for Space-Time Clustering

In a search for evidence that a disease such as leukemia is indeed an infectious disease, perhaps of viral etiology, interest will focus on whether or not the disease cases occur in clusters. In this case, a cluster will constitute a group of cases that are close both in space and time, which is called *space-time clustering* or *space-time*

Table 7.1 Kaposi's sarcoma in the West Nile district of Uganda. Locations of the homes and the date of onset of the 22 patients (data from McHardy *et al.*, 1984).

	Coordinates (km)		
Case No.	Eastings	Northings	Date of onset
1	266.8	334.3	1958
2	304.4	379.3	1959
3	265.5	315.0	1960
4	265.0	314.0	1960
5	264.2	323.0	1962
6	288.7	265.2	1962
7	290.2	294.3	1964
8	265.6	318.2	1964
9	263.7	344.4	1965
10	271.3	333.5	1966
11	267.4	344.4	1968
12	267.4	344.4	1968
13	276.5	344.6	1968
14	260.2	358.2	1971
15	264.0	296.8	1972
16	263.8	344.3	1972
17	300.5	373.0	1972
18	270.8	326.1	1973
19	258.7	344.8	1974
20	282.7	322.3	1974
21	265.3	314.9	1974
22	285.3	261.0	1974

T. Tango, *Statistical Methods for Disease Clustering*,
Statistics for Biology and Health, DOI 10.1007/978-1-4419-1572-6_7,
© Springer Science+Business Media, LLC 2010

interaction and is illustrated by the following example.

Example 1

Table 7.1 shows grid coordinates of homes and the year of onset for 22 cases of Kaposi's sarcoma in the West Nile district of Uganda in 1958–1974 (McHardy *et al.*, 1984). Does this set of data suggest any evidence for space-time clustering or interaction?

7.1 Data

To test for space-time clustering, we need to collect data retrospectively on the *time of occurrence* and the *location* of each case for a defined geographic region during a specified study period. Throughout this chapter, it is assumed that:

1. we have n cases,
2. we observe a set of observed times $\{t_1, t_2, \ldots, t_n\}$,
3. A set of observed locations $\{(x_1, y_1), (x_2, y_2), \ldots, (x_n, y_n)\}$ are available within a study region, and
4. let d_{ij}^S and d_{ij}^T denote the spatial distance and time distance, respectively, and be given by

$$d_{ij}^S = \sqrt{(x_i - x_j)^2 + (y_i - y_j)^2} \tag{7.1}$$

$$d_{ij}^T = |t_i - t_j| \tag{7.2}$$

7.2 Null Hypothesis vs Alternative Hypothesis

The null hypothesis of *no space-time clustering* and the alternative hypothesis are stated as the following:

> H_0 : the times of onset (or diagnosis) of the disease under study
>
>   are randomly distributed across the case residence $\tag{7.3}$
>
> H_1 : not H_0

The null hypothesis above can be restated as follows:

> H_0 : the temporal distances between pairs of cases are independent
>
>   of the spatial distances between pairs of cases $\tag{7.4}$

7.3 Historical Overview of Methods

(It should be noted that there are several other proposed methods not mentioned here. Furthermore, readers who are not interested in the history can skip this section.)

The most widely used test for space-time clustering is the Knox test (1964a, 1964b) , which is indicated by an excess of cases that are close both in space and time. Since the mid-1960s, the Knox test has been utilized to explore space-time clustering of several cancers, such as childhood leukemia (for example, Knox, 1964b; Meighan and Knox, 1965; Till *et al.*, 1967; Mainwaring, 1966; Gunz and Spears, 1968; Glass and Mantel, 1969; Klauber and Mustacchi, 1970; Alperovitch *et al.*, 1974; Smith *et al.*, 1976; Van Steensel-Moll *et al.*, 1983; Gilman and Knox, 1991; Alexander, 1992; Petridou *et al.*, 1996), Hodgkin's disease (Alderson and Nayak, 1971; Kryscio *et al.*, 1973; Chen, Mantel, and Klingberg, 1984) and Burkitt's lymphoma (Doll, 1978). It has also been applied to other diseases such as limb defects (Lloyd and Roberts, 1973) and neural tube defects (Roberts, Laurence and Lloyd, 1975) and Kaposi's sarcoma (McHardy et al., 1984).

To apply this test, the critical space and time limits δ_1 and δ_2 that define "closeness" must be chosen *a priori* and a 2 x 2 contingency table is formed by classifying the $n(n-1)/2$ pairs of cases as close in space and time, close in space only, close in time only, or close in neither space nor time. To express the test statistic T, the observed number of pairs close in both space and time, it is convenient to define the measure of closeness in space a_{ij}^S and in time a_{ij}^T as follows:

$$a_{ij}^S = \begin{cases} 1, & i \neq j \text{ and } d_{ij}^S < \delta_1 \text{ (km)} \\ 0, & \text{otherwise} \end{cases} \tag{7.5}$$

$$\tag{7.6}$$

$$a_{ij}^T = \begin{cases} 1, & i \neq j \text{ and } d_{ij}^T < \delta_2 \text{ (days)} \\ 0, & \text{otherwise} \end{cases} \tag{7.7}$$

This type of measure of closeness is intended to detect "hot-spot" clustering. Then it is shown that

$$T = \frac{1}{2} \sum_{i=1}^{n} \sum_{j=1}^{n} a_{ij}^S a_{ij}^T \tag{7.8}$$

Knox considered that T could be approximately Poisson in the limit of small expectation, although pairs are dependent. In his example of 96 cases of childhood leukemia, giving rise to 4560 pairs, there are 152 close pairs in time (less than 60 days) and 25 close pairs in space (within 1 km) for a total expectation of 0.83 ($= 152 \times 25/4560$) pairs, close both in space and time (Table 7.2). The observed number of close pairs, five, is highly significant using Poisson approximation,

Table 7.2 96 cases of childhood leukemia in Northumberland and Durham, U.K. (Knox, 1964).

	Space		
	(< 1km)	(≥ 1km)	Total
Time (< 60 days)	5	147	152
(≥ 60 days)	20	4388	4408
Total	25	4535	4560

$$p = 1 - \sum_{k=1}^{4} \frac{0.83^k}{k!} \exp(-0.83) = 0.0017$$

Barton and David (1966) showed that, although use of the Poisson approximation is appropriate in some situations, in general it could yield misleading results. Barton and David (1966) and Mantel (1967) developed more valid permutation variance.

Pinkel and Nefzger (1959) proposed a cell-occupancy approach to test for space-time clustering. Assuming that r cases are randomly allocated to m space-time cells with uniform population density, these investigators developed an exact test for determining the probability of observing k cases close both in space and in time. However, the uniform population assumption was too impractical.

Barton, David, and Herrington (1965) and David and Barton (1966) developed a test analogous to analysis of variance, involving the ratio of within-group variance to overall variance. Pairs of cases close in time are formed into time clusters and then the test statistic is the ratio of the average squared geographic distance between cases within time clusters to the average squared distance between all cases. Under the null hypothesis of no space-time interaction, one would expect this ratio to be 1. When clustering is present, this ratio is smaller than 1. To assess significance, David and Barton suggested using a randomization test to determine the exact distribution of this ratio. One practical weakness of the test is that the small distances, which are of most interest, have less influence on the statistic than the large distances. In fact, the large distances may so dominate the statistic that they mask any clustering. The other weakness is that clusters occurring in different areas but overlapping in time will distort the analysis. When applied to Knox's original childhood data, the test failed to corroborate Knox's result. Pinkel, Dawd and Bross (1963), in a similar approach, interchanged the roles of space and time.

Mantel (1967) developed a generalization of the Knox test in the sense that Knox's test can be derived as a special case of Mantel's test. This test has also been applied to space-time clustering of childhood leukemia (for example, Klauber, 1968; Glass and Mantel, 1969; Klauber and Mustacchi, 1970; Glass et al., 1971; Alperovitch et al., 1974) along with the Knox test, and the property of the test has been studied by many statisticians. The test statistic is the sum over all pairs of cases of a function of the distance between two cases multiplied by a function of the time between two cases. Mantel recommended using reciprocal transformations of the distances to increase the influence of close distances and decrease the influence of long distances. Mantel (1967) and Siemiatycki (1978) concluded that the test has low power if no transformation is made. A constant must be added to the distances before making the reciprocal transformation because of the possibility of very small or zero time and/or space distances. Therefore, the test statistic is given by the same form (7.8), where

$$a_{ij}^S = \frac{1}{d_{ij}^S + c_1} \tag{7.9}$$

$$a_{ij}^T = \frac{1}{d_{ij}^T + c_2} \tag{7.10}$$

This type of measure of closeness is intended to detect so-called "clinal" clustering that has a monotone decrease in disease risk as distance increases. Unfortunately, the constants c_1, c_2 chosen influence the value of the test statistic and the outcome of the test of significance. Mantel suggested that, for best results, *the constants be close to the expected distances between close pairs*. However, the rationale for this seems to be unclear. Mantel also indicated a possibility that, for large n, T may be approximately normally distributed. However, Klauber (1971) and Siemiatycki (1978) found the distribution of T to be highly skewed and showed that although the use of the normal approximation is appropriate when T is highly significant or non-significant, its use is inappropriate when T has borderline significance. Siemiatycki (1978) fitted a standard Pearson probability distribution to Mantel's T by calculating the third and fourth moments and showed this approximation to be better than the normal approximation. Therefore, practically, a test of statistical significance is obtained by obtaining the exact randomization distribution of Mantel's T or by using Monte Carlo simulation to obtain an approximation to the distribution of T. Although Mantel generalizes the Knox test using actual space and time distances by avoiding arbitrary space and time critical limits, the test statistic also has arbitrary constants and the proposed normal approximation is poor.

On the other hand, Pike and Smith (1968) also generalized Knox's test by taking the subject's likely movements in space during susceptible and infectious latent periods into account. Pairs of cases are considered close in space if their geographic areas of infectivity and susceptibility overlap, and close in time if their periods of infectivity and susceptibility overlap. The test statistic is the number of pairs close in both space and time.

Lloyd and Roberts (1973) considered a test for either spatial or temporal clustering using the number of pairs among all possible pairs of cases that are close in space (or in time) as the test statistic. Their test was applied for the 57 cases of congenital limb defects diagnosed in singleton births in Cardiff in 1964–67. For comparison, they took five control samples, each of size 57, drawn at random from the list of all singleton births in Cardiff during the same time period (Table 7.3). Smith and Pike (1974) noted that their test can be viewed as a special case of Knox's test. Let each of the n cases have onset on day 0 and the m controls have onsets on days $1, 2, ..., m$, respectively. The number of close pairs is then in the form of a Knox test if the critical time distance is defined as zero. Then, the randomization of times of onset is exactly equivalent to randomly selecting n persons from $n + m$ and counting the

Table 7.3 Frequency distribution of all possible pairs (limb defects and random samples) by distance (Lloyd and Roberts, 1973).

	Distance in 100 meters (d)						
	$d < 1$	$1 \le d < 2$	$2 \le d < 3$	$3 \le d < 4$	$4 \le d < 10$	$10 \le d$	Total
Limb cases	5	11	12	12	73	1483	1596
Sample 1	6	4	4	12	97	1473	1596
Sample 2	2	5	8	10	106	1465	1596
Sample 3	5	7	8	6	115	1455	1596
Sample 4	2	5	6	16	76	1491	1596
Sample 5	0	5	4	11	117	1459	1596

number of pairs close in space. They also suggested that matched controls be used in the procedure.

Tests related to the Knox test have unknown parameters δ_1 and δ_2, and Mantel's procedure also has unknown parameters c_1 and c_2, which leads to multiple testing by choosing a number of plausible values for these parameters. Adjustment for multiple testing is rare in the literature. For example, Tables 7.4 and 7.5 show a part of the results of the analysis (Glass and Mantel, 1969) of 298 in childhood leukemia deaths Los Angeles during 1960–1964. Glass and Mantel reported a total of 48 analyses by the Knox test, employing eight different critical space limits δ_1 and six critical time limits δ_2, and reported a total of 60 analyses by the Mantel test using ten different space constants c_1 and six different time constants c_2. However, most of the standardized test statistics Z are negative, indicating no suggestive indication of space-time clustering. To deal with the multiplicity of critical limits, Baker (1996) proposed maximizing the standardized T with respect to δ_1 and δ_2 in the user-specified range of sensible values (L_1, U_1) and (L_2, U_2)

$$Z_{\max} = \sup_{\delta_1, \delta_2} \frac{T(\delta_1, \delta_2) - \mu(\delta_1, \delta_2)}{\sigma(\delta_1, \delta_2)} \qquad (7.11)$$

where μ and σ^2 are the permutation mean and variance of T. To find the distribution of the test statistic under the null hypothesis, Monte Carlo hypothesis testing is required. Baker gave some justification of this procedure, which comes from the statistical theory that the likelihood ratio test is asymptotically equivalent to the score test for a local alternative. Furthermore, he showed that the values of the unknown (nuisance) parameters that maximize the test statistic are the maximum likelihood estimators. This procedure will work for any choice of measures of closeness a_{ij}^S and a_{ij}^T.

Chen, Mantel, and Klingberg (1984) compared the powers of three tests, Knox, Mantel, and Ederer-Myers-Mantel, by applying them to simulated data. The simulated data corresponded to three alternative nonnull models for the distribution, transmission, and development of Hodgkin's disease (HD) that were formulated in

Table 7.4 298 childhood leukemia deaths in Los Angeles County during, 1960–1964 using the Knox approach. Part of the results in Table 1 of Glass and Mantel (1969) are reproduced.

Critical space limit δ_1 (km)		Critical time limit δ_2 (months)					Total
		≤ 0.5	≤ 1	≤ 2	≤ 4	≤ 6	
≤ 0.53	Pairs	0	1	2	2	2	10
	Expected	0.17	0.51	0.82	1.42	1.99	
	Z	–0.42	0.71	1.36	0.53	0.01	
≤ 1.06	Pairs	1	2	5	11	16	65
	Expected	1.14	3.29	5.33	9.21	13.00	
	Z	–0.13	–0.73	–0.15	0.64	0.95	
≤ 1.58	Pairs	2	6	9	19	29	145
	Expected	2.54	7.34	11.90	20.53	28.90	
	Z	–0.34	0.51	–0.88	–0.37	0.02	
≤ 2.20	Pairs	3	9	13	29	44	243
	Expected	4.25	12.31	19.94	4.41	48.43	
	Z	–0.61	–0.97	–1.63	–1.00	–0.71	
Total		774	2241	3632	6267	8819	44253

$Z = (\text{Pairs} - \text{Expected})/\sqrt{\text{Variance}}$

accordance with the results of published studies. Their results indicate that the three techniques may not be sufficiently sensitive to the clustering in a real data set of HD cases. They concluded that the inconclusive results obtained to date with regard to the clustering of HD may be related to the low power of the statistical techniques employed. Wartenberg and Greenberg (1990) compared the powers of the Ederer-Myers-Mantel and Mantel tests and concluded that both tests fail to detect clustering when it actually exists.

Jacquez (1996) gave several reasons why the Knox and Mantel tests have a low ability to detect disease clusters. One reason was that selection of critical limits for Knox's test, and of an appropriate data transformation for Mantel's test, is subjective. This problem, however, can be resolved by Baker's approach. A more essential reason is that the Knox space critical limit is invariant with changing population density, which might be unreasonable because the distance between cases will decrease when the background population density increases. That is, geographic distance is not always an appropriate measure of spatial proximity, and instead nearest neighbor relationships seem a logical alternative. Based on these ideas, Jacquez (1996) proposed a different Knox-type test statistic $T = (T_k)$, where the measures of closeness is defined by the k nearest neighbors (abbreviated k NN) such that

Table 7.5 298 childhood leukemia deaths in Los Angeles County during 1960–1964 using the Mantel approach. Part of the results in Table 2 of Glass and Mantel (1969) are reproduced.

Space		Time constants c_2 (months)					
constants c_1(km)		0.5	1	2	4	6	12
0.09	Observed T	279.57	221.40	174.51	133.37	111.54	78.46
	$E(T)$	285.14	224.58	176.34	134.42	112.29	78.84
	Z	−1.08	−1.01	−1.09	−1.09	−1.10	−1.08
0.18	Observed T	275.50	218.07	171.84	131.30	109.79	77.20
	$E(T)$	280.31	220.77	173.35	132.14	110.38	77.53
	Z	−1.17	−1.17	−1.13	−1.08	−1.08	−1.12
0.26	Observed T	271.99	215.24	169.59	129.56	108.33	76.17
	$E(T)$	276.40	217.74	170.97	130.33	108.87	76.46
	Z	−1.21	−1.21	−1.14	−1.09	−1.08	−1.10
0.35	Observed T	268.83	212.70	167.56	128.00	107.02	75.25
	$E(T)$	273.06	215.06	168.87	128.72	107.53	75.52
	Z	−1.23	−1.23	−1.16	−1.10	−1.08	−1.09

Z: Standardized T or $(T - E(T))/\sqrt{\mathrm{Var}(T)}$.

$$a_{ij}^S = \begin{cases} 1, & \text{if case } j \text{ is a } k \text{ NN of case } i \text{ in space} \\ 0, & \text{otherwise} \end{cases} \tag{7.12}$$

$$a_{ij}^T = \begin{cases} 1, & \text{if case } j \text{ is a } k \text{ NN of case } i \text{ in time} \\ 0, & \text{otherwise} \end{cases} \tag{7.13}$$

Jacquez insisted that this procedure does not require parameters such as critical distances to be estimated from data. However, this procedure also faces multiple testing by repeating tests for many values of k. For this problem, Jacquez considered a kind of artificial measure called *centroid distance* to combine probabilities across levels of $k = 1, 2, ..., m$. For power comparisons, Jacquez devised a four-state Markov HIV model under realistic population distributions and showed that the k-NN test has superior performance relative to the Knox and Mantel tests. However, the infectious process in his simulation model was based on a "nearest-neighbour mechanism". It seems to me that the k-NN approach is not always superior to geographical distance in detecting space-time clustering because the k-NN approach gives equal weight to all the nearest neighbors even though there are some cases situated far apart from each other, which may cause an apparent statistically significant clustering.

Diggle *et al.* (1995) extends the second-order methods for spatial clustering (Diggle and Chetwynd, 1991) to detect space-time clustering in point process data, which is closely related to Knox's test statistic. Diggle *et al.* (1995) define the K-function in space and time as follows:

$$K(s,t) = E[\text{number of further events occurring within}$$
$$\text{distance } s \text{ and time } t \text{ of an arbitrary event}]/\lambda$$

where λ indicates the intensity representing the expected number of events per unit space and unit time. Let $\{(x_i, y_i, t_i) : i = 1, ..., n\}$ denote the locations and times of all events within a spatial-temporal region $A \times (0, T)$. Then an approximately unbiased estimator for $K(s,t)$ is

$$\hat{K}(s,t) = \frac{|A| T}{n(n-1)} \sum_{i=1}^{n} \sum_{j=1, i \neq j}^{n} w_{ij} v_{ij} I(d_{ij}^S \leq s) I(d_{ij}^T \leq t)$$

where $I(\cdot)$ denotes the indicator function and w_{ij} and v_{ij} constitute a correction for edge effects in estimating second-order properties in space and time, respectively. w_{ij} is calculated as the reciprocal of the proportion of the circumference of the circle with center (x_i, y_j) and radius d_{ij}^S that lies within A and $v_{ij} = 1$ if both ends of the interval of length $2d_{ij}^T$ and center t_i lie within $(0, T)$, $v_{ij} = 2$, otherwise.

In Section 2.2, I have already explained that there is no need for edge correction for testing the null hypothesis of no clustering in the study of disease clustering. Namely, if we set all $w_{ij} = 1$ and all $v_{ij} = 1$, then the K-function above is equivalent to Knox's test statistic for spatial and temporal threshold separations s and t. However, Diggle et al. provided the user with several useful tools to examine space-time clustering. For a spatial-temporal Poisson process in which the spatial and temporal components are independent, the K-function factorizes as

$$K(s,t) = K_1(s)_2K(t)$$

where $K_1(s)$ and $K_2(t)$ are the K-functions of the spatial and temporal component processes. Then, Diggle et al. (1995) define the three functions as the diagnostics for space-time interactions:

$$D(s,t) = K(s,t) - K_1(s)K_2(t)$$
$$R(s,t) = \hat{D}(s,t)/\sqrt{\text{Var}(\hat{D}(s,t))}$$
$$D_0(s,t) = D(s,t)/\{K_1(s)K_2(t)\} = K(s,t)/\{K_1(s)K_2(t)\} - 1$$

A perspective plot of the surface $\hat{D}(s,t)$ gives information on the scale and pattern of the dependence between spatial and temporal components and $R(s,t)$ are standardized residuals. The function $\hat{D}_0(s,t)$ denotes the proportional increase or excess risk attributable to space-time interactions. Then, as a test statistic for space-time interaction, Diggle et al. (1995) propose a summation of standardized residuals over a predefined discrete set of equally spaced spatial distance s_k, $k = 1, ..., m_s$, and equally spaced temporal distance t_j, $j = 1, ..., m_t$:

$$U_{\text{sum}} = \sum_{k=1}^{m_s} \sum_{j=1}^{m_t} R(s_k, t_j)$$

Table 7.6 Number of pairs by space and time distances between nuclear explosions and earthquakes in Nevada. (Klauber, 1971).

	Space		
	(< 100 km)	(≥ 100 km)	Total
Time (< 24 hours)	9	3	12
(≥ 24 hours)	399	745	748
Total	408	1144	1156

However, it seems to me that the followng Max test rather than the Sum test would be more powerful for detecting space-time interactions:

$$U_{\max} = \max_{k=1,\dots,m_s, j=1,\dots,m_t} R(s_k, t_j)$$

To find the distribution of the test statistic under the null hypothesis, Monte Carlo hypothesis testing by permuting the times among the fixed spatial locations is required here also.

Pike and Smith (1974) proposed a case-control version of tests for space-time clustering using information from a set of matched control persons as well as the cases themselves. The case-control approach attempts to examine whether cases under study have had more relevant contact with each other than have a suitably chosen control group. The test statistic is

$$T = \frac{1}{2} \sum_{i=1}^{n} \sum_{j=1}^{n} a_{ij}^S a_{ij}^T$$

which is the same form as that of the Knox test (7.8). However, the null distribution is different. In the case-control study, the null distribution is obtained by selecting n persons from the total $2n$ persons, where we take one person at random from each pair (either a case or a control) and calculate T. There are 2^n possible different random selections, and the p-values of the observed values of T can be obtained by the exact permutational approach or Monte Carlo hypothesis testing. Jacquez (1996) also considered a case-control version based on the k-NN approach.

Tests for space-time clustering have been extended to the two-sample problem by Klauber (1971). In the two-sample problem, one is concerned with two different data sets, A and B, of distinguishable points having space coordinates and time coordinates, and one may wish to hypothesize that two different sets of diseases may be the result of the same contagious disease. Therefore, the purpose of two-sample tests for space-time clustering is to test whether or not there is a tendency for pairs of cases, one from A and one from B, to be close both in space and time. Let (x_{Ai}, y_{Ai}, t_{Ai}), $i = 1,\dots,n_A$ and (x_{Bi}, y_{Bi}, t_{Bi}), $i = 1,\dots,n_B$ denote the space and time coordinates of two sets of point observations, A and B, respectively, in a given region and time interval. Let a_{ij}^S and a_{ij}^T here be real-valued functions of the space and time distances

$$d_{ij}^S = \sqrt{(x_{Ai} - x_{Bj})^2 + (y_{Ai} - y_{Bj})^2}$$

$$d_{ij}^T = |t_{Ai} - t_{Bj}|$$

between case i from A and case j from B, where a Knox-type function or Mantel-type function can be used. Then the test statistic is again of the same form:

$$T = \frac{1}{2} \sum_{i=1}^{n_A} \sum_{j=1}^{n_B} a_{ij}^S a_{ij}^T.$$

The null distribution of T is a randomization distribution randomly permuting the coordinates of one of the sets while the other is fixed. Klauber illustrated his test with data from the 17 nuclear tests that took place at the Nevada Test Site (assumed fixed) and the 68 earthquakes (assumed random) that occurred within a 400 km radius of the Test Site during the first six months of 1968. The data are summarized in Table 7.6. The observed values are $T = 9$ and $E(T) = 4.24$. As the normality assumption is poor, Klauber applied Monte Carlo hypothesis testing with 500 replicates and obtained a p-value less than $1/500 = 0.002$. Klauber (1975) considered the case with more than two samples.

The tests described so far might indicate evidence of disease clustering in space and in time but do not directly relate consecutive observations to the clustering tendency of previous events. To cope with this problem, Lawson and Viel (1995) proposed a test that accounts for the spatial cluster structure by using directional information contained in the polar coordinate representation of the time sequence of events.

So far, we have implicitly assumed that the rate of population growth is common to all regions under study. However, it has been known that tests for space-time interactions are biased when there are varying population growth rates in different regions. To reduce this bias, Klauber and Mustacchi (1970) suggested dividing the study period into several subperiods where the population would be stable. A test statistic is then calculated separately for each subperiod and then summed to get an overall test statistic. This surely will reduce the bias but also reduce the power of the test because pairs of cases falling in different subperiods are no longer taken into account. Kulldorff and Hjalmars (1999) examined the size of this bias of the Knox test for real data and proposed a Monte Carlo method to obtain an unbiased version of the Knox test by using the underlying population and its temporal trend aggregated to regions such as census tracts and counties over the study period. However, as most tests for space-time clustering utilize case point data, $(x_i, y_i, t_i), i = 1, ..., n$, not regional count data, a problem arises: What is the population growth rate for each case? Or can we apply the rate of population growth of the region in which the case is located?

7.4 Selected Methods

In this section, we shall describe the details of tests for space-time interaction, which are selected in terms of *widely known and/or widely used tests* in the literature.

7.4.1 Knox's Test

Goal: To count the observed number of pairs of cases close in both space and time and evaluate the significance. A significantly large number would indicate evidence of space-time clustering of the disease under study.
Null hypothesis H_0: (7.4)
Alternative hypothesis H_1: not H_0

Test statistic

The Knox test statistic is

$$T = \frac{1}{2} \sum_{i=1}^{n} \sum_{j=1}^{n} a_{ij}^S a_{ij}^T \tag{7.14}$$

where a_{ij}^S and a_{ij}^T denote the *hot-spot type measure of closeness* in space and in time, respectively, are given by

$$a_{ij}^S = \begin{cases} 1, & i \neq j \text{ and } d_{ij}^S < \delta_1 \text{ (km)} \\ 0, & \text{otherwise} \end{cases} \tag{7.15}$$

$$a_{ij}^T = \begin{cases} 1, & i \neq j \text{ and } d_{ij}^T < \delta_2 \text{ (days)} \\ 0, & \text{otherwise} \end{cases} \tag{7.16}$$

and δ_1 and δ_2 are unknown critical space and time limits and have to be prespecified by the user. Barton and David (1966) derived the exact formula for the variance of T

$$E(T) = \frac{N_{1s}N_{1t}}{N} \tag{7.17}$$

$$V(T) = \frac{N_{1s}N_{1t}}{N} + \frac{4N_{2s}N_{2t}}{n(n-1)(n-2)} - \left(\frac{N_{1s}N_{1t}}{N}\right)^2$$
$$+ \frac{4\{N_{1s}(N_{1s}-1) - N_{2s}\}\{N_{1t}(N_{1t}-1) - N_{2t}\}}{n(n-1)(n-2)(n-3)} \tag{7.18}$$

where

$$N = \frac{n(n-1)}{2}, \; N_{1s} = \frac{1}{2}\sum_{i=1}^{n}\sum_{j=1}^{n}a_{ij}^{S}, \; N_{1t} = \frac{1}{2}\sum_{i=1}^{n}\sum_{j=1}^{n}a_{ij}^{T}$$

$$N_{2s} = \frac{1}{2}\sum_{i=1}^{n}\sum_{j=1}^{n}\sum_{k\neq j}a_{ij}^{S}a_{ik}^{S}, \; N_{2t} = \frac{1}{2}\sum_{i=1}^{n}\sum_{j=1}^{n}\sum_{k\neq j}a_{ij}^{T}a_{ik}^{T}$$

where N_{2s} denotes the number of times two case pairs close in space are contiguous and N_{2s} is defined similarly for time.

Null distribution

Given values of these two parameters δ_1, δ_2 and the observed values $T = t$, the null distribution of T or its p-value can be approximated by either one of the following,

1. Poisson distribution when N_{1t} and N_{1s} are small compared with N:

$$p\text{-value} = 1 - \sum_{k=0}^{t-1}\frac{E(T)^k}{k!}\exp\{-E(T)\} \tag{7.19}$$

or mid-p-value

$$p\text{-value} = 1 - \sum_{k=0}^{t}\frac{E(T)^k}{k!}\exp\{-E(T)\} + \frac{1}{2}\frac{E(T)^t}{t!}\exp\{-E(T)\} \tag{7.20}$$

2. Normal distribution with mean and variance derived by Barton and David (1966)

$$p\text{-value} = 1 - \Phi\left(\frac{t - E(T)}{\sqrt{V(T)}}\right) \tag{7.21}$$

where $\Phi(.)$ denotes the standard normal distribution function.
3. Monte Carlo hypothesis testing by permuting the times (spatial locations) among the fixed spatial locations (times) can be carried out to obtain the null distribution of T and the Monte Carlo simulated p-value (2.17).

7.4.2 Mantel's Test

Goal: To calculate the sum, over all pairs of cases, of a measure of closeness in space multiplied by a measure of closeness in time, which includes the Knox test statistic as a special case, and evaluate its significance. A significantly large value would indicate evidence of space-time clustering of the disease under study.
Null hypothesis H_0: (7.4)
Alternative hypothesis H_1: not H_0

Test statistic

The Mantel test statistic is

$$T = \frac{1}{2} \sum_{i=1}^{n} \sum_{j=1}^{n} a_{ij}^{S} a_{ij}^{T} \tag{7.22}$$

where a_{ij}^{S} and a_{ij}^{T} denote the *clinal type measures of closeness* in space and in time, respectively, and are given by

$$a_{ij}^{S} = \frac{1}{d_{ij}^{S} + c_1} \quad (a_{ii}^{S} = 0) \tag{7.23}$$

$$a_{ij}^{T} = \frac{1}{d_{ij}^{T} + c_2} \quad (a_{ii}^{T} = 0) \tag{7.24}$$

and c_1 and c_2 are unknown parameters and have to be prespecified by the user. The expected value of T is given by (7.17).

Null distribution

Given values of these two parameters, c_1 and c_2, Monte Carlo hypothesis testing by permuting the times (spatial locations) among the fixed spatial locations (times) is required to obtain the null distribution of T and the simulated p-value (2.17).

7.4.3 Baker's Max Test for the Knox Test

Baker's Max test is applicable to any tests for space-time clustering with unknown parameters to adjust for multiple testing and it is basically computer-intensive but fairly simple to program.

Goal: To find the maximum of the standardized T for the Knox test over the values δ_1, δ_2 within the user-specified range of sensible values (L_1, L_2) and (U_1, U_2), respectively, and evaluate its significance. This procedure is devised for adjusting multiple testing by choosing a number of plausible values for (δ_1, δ_2). A significantly large value would indicate evidence of space-time clustering of the disease under study.

Null hypothesis H_0: (7.4)

Alternative hypothesis H_1: not H_0

An algorithm (multiple hypothesis testing procedure)

1. Set the range (L_1, U_1) and (L_2, U_2) for space and time critical limits δ_1 and δ_2 and the number of values in the ranges to be sampled.
2. Generate N_{rep} random data sets based on random permutation $p(1), ..., p(n)$ of integers $1, ..., n$ for time.

3. For the observed data and random data sets and for each set of values of critical limits, calculate the following standardized test statistic Z for each set of value

$$Z = \frac{T - E(T)}{\sqrt{V(T)}}$$

where, for each of the random data sets,

$$T = \frac{1}{2} \sum_{i=1}^{n} \sum_{j=1}^{n} a_{ij}^S a_{p(i)p(j)}^T$$

and $E(T)$ is given by (7.17). Regarding the variance $V(T)$ for Knox's test, we can use Barton and David's formula (7.18). In general, we use the following simulated permutation variance:

(i) $SS = 0$

(ii) for each of N_{rep} random data sets, calculate

$$D = \frac{1}{2} \sum_{i=1}^{n} \sum_{j=1}^{n} a_{ij}^S a_{p(i)p(j)}^T - E(T)$$

(iii) $SS = SS + D^2$ and go to step (ii).

In the end, $V(T)$ is estimated as SS/N_{rep}.

4. For each data set, select the maximum value of Z over all sets of critical limits and let $M = \max_{\delta_1, \delta_2} Z$.

5. Suppose M_{obs} denotes the Max test statistic for the data observed and $M_1 \leq M_2 \leq \cdots \leq M_{N_{rep}}$ denotes the Max test statistic for the random data sets. Then, we have

$$p\text{-value} = \frac{R}{N_{rep} + 1} \tag{7.25}$$

where R denotes the rank of the observed test statistic M_{obs} for the data set consisting of $N_{rep} + 1$ Max test statistics.

7.4.4 Jacquez's k-NN Test

Goal: To count the observed number of pairs of cases close in both space and time, where the measure of closeness is defined by the k nearest neighbors, and evaluate its significance. A significantly large number would indicate evidence of space-time clustering of the disease under study.

Null hypothesis H_0: (7.4)

Alternative hypothesis H_1: not H_0

Test statistic

Jacquez's k-NN test statistic $T(=T_k)$ is

$$T_k = \frac{1}{2} \sum_{i=1}^{n} \sum_{j=1}^{n} a_{ij}^S a_{ij}^T \qquad (7.26)$$

where a_{ij}^S and a_{ij}^T denote the *measures of closeness* in space and in time, respectively, and are given by

$$a_{ij}^S = \begin{cases} 1, & \text{if case } j \text{ is a } k \text{ NN of case } i(\neq j) \text{ in space} \\ 0, & \text{otherwise} \end{cases} \qquad (7.27)$$

$$a_{ij}^T = \begin{cases} 1, & \text{if case } j \text{ is a } k \text{ NN of case } i(\neq j) \text{ in time} \\ 0, & \text{otherwise} \end{cases} \qquad (7.28)$$

Null distribution

Given values of k, Monte Carlo hypothesis testing by permuting the times (spatial locations) among the fixed spatial locations (times) is required to obtain the null distribution of T and the Monte Carlo simulated p-value (2.17).

Adjustment for multiple testing

Using the idea used in Tango's index (5.13, 6.20), which is similar to Baker's, the MIN test

$$P_{\min} = \min_{k=1,2,\ldots,m} \Pr\{T_k \geq t_k\} \qquad (7.29)$$

, where t_k is the observed test statistic T_k, could be a promising procedure. . The p-value of $P_{\min}$ is also obtained by Monte Carlo hypothesis testing.

7.4.5 *Diggle* et al.'s Test

Diggle *et al.*'s test statistic without edge correction is equivalent to Knox's test statistic. However, their procedure provides the user with several diagnostics useful for space-time interactions and tests to avoid multiple testing.

Goal: To calculate the difference between the K-function *in space and time* and the product of the K-function *in space* and that *in time* and evaluate the significance of difference. A significantly positive value would indicate evidence of spatial clustering of the disease under study.
Null hypothesis H_0: (7.4)
Alternative hypothesis H_1: not H_0

Test statistic

Before applying this test, the study region A and time period $[0, T]$ covering n data points must be defined and the area of the study region, $|A|$, must be calculated. Although I have already explained in Section 2.2 that there is no need for edge correction for testing the null hypothesis of no clustering in the study of disease clustering, Diggle *et al.*'s original procedure with the edge correction is described here in honor of the authors. Let

$$D(s,t) = K(s,t) - K_1(s)K_2(t) \tag{7.30}$$

where $K(s,t)$ is a K-function in space and time, which is defined as

$$K(s,t) = E[\text{number of further events occurring within}$$
$$\text{distance } s \text{ and time } t \text{ of an arbitrary event}]/\lambda$$

and $K_1(s)$ and $K_2(t)$ denote the K-function in space and in time, respectively. Then the proposed test statistic is the summation of standardized residuals over a pre-defined discrete set of equally spaced spatial distance s_k, $k = 1, ..., m_s$ and of equally spaced temporal distance t_j, $j = 1, ..., m_t$:

$$U_{\text{sum}} = \sum_{k=1}^{m_s} \sum_{j=1}^{m_t} R(s_k, t_j) = \sum_{k=1}^{m_s} \sum_{j=1}^{m_t} \hat{D}(s,t)/\sqrt{\text{Var}(\hat{D}(s,t))} \tag{7.31}$$

However, it seems to me that the following Max test is also a useful test statistic and could be more powerful than the Sum test for detecting space-time interactions in many situations:

$$U_{\text{max}} = \max_{k=1,...,m_s, j=1,...,m_t} R(s_k, t_j) \tag{7.32}$$

where

$$\hat{K}(s,t) = \frac{|A| T}{n(n-1)} \sum_{i=1}^{n} \sum_{j=1, i \neq j}^{n} w_{ij} v_{ij} I(d_{ij}^S \leq s) I(d_{ij}^T \leq t) \tag{7.33}$$

w_{ij} : the reciprocal of the proportion of the circumference of the circle with center (x_i, y_j) and radius d_{ij}^S that lies within A

v_{ij} : $=1$, if both ends of the interval of length $2d_{ij}^T$ and center t_i lie within $(0, T)$; $= 2$, otherwise.

$$\text{Var}(\hat{D}(s,t)) = \frac{|A|^2 T^2}{n(n-1)} \Big\{ (W_1^2 - 4W_2 + 2W_3)(V_1^2 - 4V_2 + 2V_3)/n^{(4)}$$
$$+ 4(W_2 - W_3)(V_2 - V_3)/n^{(3)} + 2W_3 V_3/n^{(2)} - W_1^2 V_1^2/(n^{(2)})^2 \Big\} \tag{7.34}$$

$$n^{(r)} = n(n-1)\cdots(n-r+1)$$

$$W_1 = \sum_{i=1}^{n}\sum_{j=1}^{n}(w_{ij}+w_{ji})I(d_{ij}^S \leq s)/2 = \sum_{i=1}^{n}\sum_{j=1}^{n}S_{ij}, \quad (S_{ii}=0)$$

$$W_2 = \sum_{i=1}^{n}\left(\sum_{j=1}^{n}S_{ij}\right)\left(\sum_{k=1}^{n}S_{ik}\right)$$

$$W_3 = \sum_{i=1}^{n}\sum_{j=1}^{n}S_{ij}^2$$

$$V_1 = \sum_{i=1}^{n}\sum_{j=1}^{n}(v_{ij}+v_{ji})I(d_{ij}^T \leq t)/2 = \sum_{i=1}^{n}\sum_{j=1}^{n}Z_{ij}, \quad (Z_{ii}=0)$$

$$V_2 = \sum_{i=1}^{n}\left(\sum_{j=1}^{n}Z_{ij}\right)\left(\sum_{k=1}^{n}Z_{ik}\right)$$

$$V_3 = \sum_{i=1}^{n}\sum_{j=1}^{n}Z_{ij}^2$$

Diagnostic plots

Diggle *et al.* (1995) propose the three plots as diagnostics for space-time interactions:

1. A perspective plot of the surface $\hat{D}(s,t)$, which gives information on the scale and pattern of the dependence between spatial and temporal components.
2. A perspective plot of the surface

$$\hat{D}_0(s,t) = \hat{D}(s,t)/\{K_1(s)K_2(t)\} = \hat{K}(s,t)/\{\hat{K}_1(s)\hat{K}_2(t)\} - 1 \qquad (7.35)$$

   which denotes the proportional increase or excess risk attributable to space-time interactions.
3. A plot of standardized residuals $R(s,t)$ against $\hat{K}_1(s)\hat{K}_2(t)$, analogous to a plot of standardized residuals against fitted values in regression models.

Null distribution

Monte Carlo hypothesis testing by permuting the times (spatial locations) among the fixed spatial locations (times) is required to obtain the null distribution of U_{sum} or U_{max} and the Monte Carlo simulated p-value (2.17).

Software

To apply Diggle *et al.*'s method, we can use the package **splancs**:spatial and space-time point pattern analysis (Rowlingson and Diggle, 1993), which can easily be installed in the R system. The original sources can be accessed at

http://www.maths.lancs.ac.uk/~rowlings/Splancs/.

7.4.6 Kulldorff and Hjalmars's Approach for the Knox Test

Goal: To calculate the Knox test statistic adjusted for varying population growth rates in different regions and evaluate its significance. A significantly large number would indicate evidence of space-time clustering of the disease under study.
Null hypothesis H_0: (7.4)
Alternative hypothesis H_1: not H_0

An algorithm for the adjusted Knox test

An algorithm is described as follows, where the values of critical limits δ_1 and δ_2 are given.

1. Generate N_{rep} random data sets by Monte Carlo simulation, where each replication has the same number of cases as the observed data. The location and time of each case should be random, with probability proportional to the population size for that location and time or to the expected number of cases under the null hypothesis adjusted for potential confounders such as age.
2. Calculate the test statistic T for the observed data and random data sets.
3. For each data set, normalize T using a permutation variance (7.18)

$$Z = \frac{T - E(T \mid N_{1s}, N_{1t})}{\sqrt{V(T \mid N_{1s}, N_{1t}, N_{2s}, N_{2t})}}$$

   where it should be noted that N_{1s}, N_{1t}, N_{2s}, and N_{2t} change in each simulated data set.
4. The simulated p-value is calculated as $R/(N_{\text{rep}} + 1)$ where R denotes the rank of the observed test statistic for the data set consisting of $N_{\text{rep}} + 1$ test statistics.

Adjustment for multiple testing

To adjust for multiple testing, Kulldorff and Hjalmars adopted Baker's idea:

1. Set the range (L_1, U_1) and (L_2, U_2) for space and time critical limits δ_1 and δ_2 and the number of values in the ranges to be sampled.
2. Generate N_{rep} random data sets by Monte Carlo simulation in the same way as above.
3. For the observed data and random data sets and for each set of values of critical limits, calculate the standardized test statistic Z for each set of value

$$Z = \frac{T - E(T \mid N_{1s}, N_{1t})}{\sqrt{V(T \mid N_{1s}, N_{1t}, N_{2s}, N_{2t})}}$$

4. For each data set, select the maximum value of Z over all sets of critical limits and let $M = \max_{\delta_1, \delta_2} Z$.

5. Suppose M_{obs} denotes the max test statistic for the data observed and $M_1 \leq M_2 \leq \cdots \leq M_{N_{rep}}$ denote the max test statistics for the random data sets. Then, we have

$$p\text{-value} = \frac{R}{N_{rep} + 1} \tag{7.36}$$

where R denotes the rank of the observed test statistic M_{obs} for the data set consisting of $N_{rep} + 1$ Max test statistics.

7.5 Illustrations with Real Data

In this section, some selected one-sample methods will be illustrated with a published data set from McHardy *et al.* (1984), who gave grid coordinates of homes and the year of onset for 22 cases of Kaposi's sarcoma in the West Nile district of Uganda. For illustration, let us assume here that the rate of population growth in the West Nile district was common to all regions during the study period.

7.5.1 Kaposi's Sarcoma in the West Nile Distric of Uganda

McHardy *et al.* applied the Knox (1964) and Barton and David (1966) methods to 22 Kaposi's sarcoma patients diagnosed from 1958 to 1974 in the West Nile district of Uganda. The authors state that computer analysis using these two methods did not reveal statistically significant space-time clustering. Critical time limits varied from < 1 year to < 5 years and the critical space limits from 1 km to 24 km. Grid coordinates of the homes and the date of onset of these 22 patients are listed in Table 7.1. Baker (1996) also analyzed these data using a Knox test and Baker's Max test. Baker considered the case $\delta_1 = 2$ and $\delta_2 = 0$ for the Knox test and obtained $T = 2$ and p-value = 0.0295 based upon Monte Carlo hypothesis testing with $N_{rep} = 50,000$.

First, let us apply the Knox test with the same parameter values as those of Baker, $\delta_1 = 2$ and $\delta_2 = 0$. In this case, we have $E(T) = 0.325$ and $Var(T) = 0.326$, indicating that the Poisson approximation is good. Therefore, the Poisson approximation (7.19) led to $p = 0.0426$, or its mid-p-value (7.20) is 0.0235. If we use the normal approximation (7.21), we have $p = 0.00167$, which is quite liberal because the normal approximation is poor since $E(T) = 0.325$ is so small. Output from the R function **KnoxA.test** (Appendix) with approximated p-values is shown below.

Output from the R function KnoxA.test

```
> del1< − 2; del2< − 0
> KnoxA.test(x,y,time,del1,del2)
$Knox.T:
[1] 2
$Expected:
[1] 0.3246753
$Var:
[1] 0.3260965
$Standardized:
[1] 2.933769
$Poisson.p.value:
[1] 0.04257504
$Poisson.Mid.p.value:
[1] 0.02352772
$Normal.p.value:
[1] 0.001674367
```

Next, let us carry out Monte Carlo hypothesis testing with $N_{rep} = 999$. A frequency of 999 simulated T's plus one observed $T = 2$ is shown below:

T	0	1	2	3	Total
Frequency	722	249	25	4	999

Therefore, the observed $T = 2$ is 29th largest among (999+1) T's, indicating $p = 0.029$, close to Baker's result. Output from the R program **KnoxM.test** (Appendix) for Knox's test with a Monte Carlo simulated p-value is shown below.

Output from the R program of the R function KnoxM.test

```
> Nrep< − 999
> out< − KnoxM.test(x,y,time,del1,del2,Nrep)
> table(out$Freq)
  0    1    2    3
722 249  25    4
> out$Simulated.p.value
[1] 0.029
```

Table 7.7 Knox's test with a Poisson mid-p-value for 22 patients with Kaposi's sarcoma in the West Nile district of Uganda (data from McHardy *et al.*, 1984).

Critical space limit δ_1 (km)		Critical time limit δ_2 (years)					
		0	≤ 1	≤ 2	≤ 3	≤ 4	Total
≤ 1	Pairs	1	1	1	1	1	4
	Expected	0.260	0.537	1.022	1.264	1.662	
	Poisson mid-p	0.129	0.258	0.251	0.259	0.645	
≤ 2	Pairs	2	2	2	2	2	5
	Expected	0.325	0.671	1.277	1.580	2.078	
	Poisson mid-p	0.024	0.088	0.251	0.340	0.480	
≤ 3	Pairs	2	2	2	2	2	5
	Expected	0.325	0.671	1.277	1.580	2.078	
	Poisson mid-p	0.024	0.088	0.251	0.340	0.480	
≤ 4	Pairs	2	2	2	4	7	11
	Expected	0.714	1.476	2.809	3.476	4.571	
	Poisson mid-p	0.098	0.310	0.651	0.364	0.135	
≤ 5	Pairs	2	2	2	4	8	13
	Expected	0.844	1.745	3.320	4.108	5.403	
	Poisson mid-p	0.138	0.388	0.744	0.490	0.138	
Total		15	31	59	73	96	231

Next, let us repeat a total of 25 Knox tests by using five different space limits $\delta_1 = 1, 2, 3, 4, 5$ (km) and five different time limits $\delta_2 = 0, 1, 2, 3, 4$ (years). The result is shown in Table 7.7. Results of multiple tests suggest that space-time clustering may be occurring within the same year but an appropriate critical space limit is not clear due to multiple tests.

Then, in order to adjust for multiple testing, we shall apply Baker's Max test using the same sets of critical limits. Calculation was done using Fortran code (not shown), and Baker's Max test gave (i) the observed Max test statistic is $M_{obs} = 2.933$ for $T = 2$, $\delta_1 = 2, 3$, and $\delta_2 = 0$ and (ii) adjusted p-value $p = 0.106$ with $N_{rep} = 9999$ repetitions, which is also close to Baker's result $p = 0.094$.

As the next analysis, we shall apply the Mantel test with $c_1 = 1$ and $c_2 = 1/5$ by putting more weight on the zero distance in time $d_{ij}^T = 0$. The null distribution is obtained by Monte Carlo hypothesis testing with $N_{rep} = 999$. Output from the R function **Mantel.test** (Appendix) for Mantel's test with a Monte Carlo simulated p-value is shown below.

Output from the R function Mantel.test

```
> c1 < - 1; c2 < - 1/5
> Nrep < - 999
> out < - Mantel.test(x,y,time,c1,c2,Nrep)
> hist(out$Freq)       (see Figure 7.1)
> out$Mantel.T
[1] 12.1751
> out$Simulated.p.value
[1] 0.032
>
```

The observed test statistic is $T = 12.18$, with simulated p-value $p = 0.032$. The histogram of the simulated Mantel test statistic T is shown in Figure 7.1. Table 7.8 shows a total of 36 sets of Mantel tests for six different spatial constants $c_1 = 0.1, 0.2, 0.5, 1, 2, 5$ (km) and six different time constants $c_2 = 0.1, 0.2, 0.5, 1, 2, 5$ (years). These results suggest that we can observe significant space-time clustering ($p < 0.05$) in most cells when both parameter values are less than 1.0. Next, in order to adjust for multiple testing, we shall apply Baker's Max test using the same 36 sets of critical limits. The calculation was done using Fortran code (not shown), and Baker's Max test based on the Mantel test gave a significant space-time interaction: Mantel's test statistic is $T = 116.51$ and the Max test statistic (standardized) is $M_{obs} = 3.38$ at $c_1 = 0.1$ and $c_2 = 0.1$ with adjusted p-value $p = 0.0268$.

As the next analysis, we shall apply Jacquez's k-NN test for ten different values of $k = 1, 2, ..., 10$. Due to the lack of precision for time, measured in years only, there are many artifactual "tied" temporal nearest neighbors, which may make the computation a little bit complicated. So, to avoid this, we added small uniform random numbers to values of "years" so that the number of tied nearest neighbors can be negligible. Needless to say, the results depend on the seed of random numbers to some extent, but the difference was not so large. The null distribution is again obtained by Monte Carlo hypothesis testing with $N_{rep} = 999$. Output from the R function **Jacquez.test** (Appendix) for Jacquez's test with $k = 1$ is shown below.

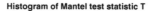

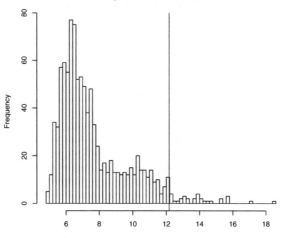

Fig. 7.1 Histogram of the simulated Mantel test statistic T based on Monte Carlo hypothesis testing with $N_{rep} = 999$ repetitions and the location of the observed Mantel test statistic.

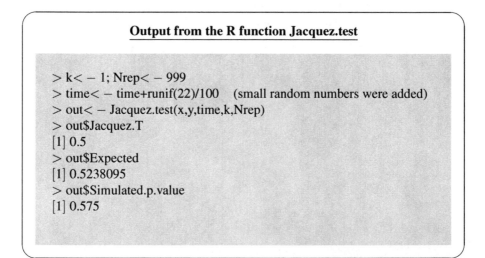

The observed test statistic is $T = 0.5$ with simulated p-value $p = 0.575$. Table 7.9 shows a total of ten sets of Jacquez test results using a fixed seed. These results suggest that Jacquez's nearest neighbors approach cannot detect space-time clustering for all values of k for these data.

As the last analysis, we shall apply Diggle *et al*'s test using the package **splancs**, where we use five different space limits $\delta_1 = 1, 2, 3, 4, 5$ (km) and five different time limits $\delta_2 = 0, 1, 2, 3, 4$ (years), which is the same setting as the application of

Table 7.8 Mantel's test with Monte Carlo p-value with $N_{rep} = 999$ for 22 patients with Kaposi's sarcoma in the West Nile district of Uganda (data from McHardy *et al.*, 1984).

Critical space limit c_1 (km)		Critical time limit c_2 (years)					
		0.1	0.2	0.5	1	2	5
0.1	T	116.51	59.90	25.73	14.08	7.96	3.87
	Expected	26.61	16.51	9.92	7.12	5.11	3.10
	Monte Carlo p	0.022	0.025	0.035	0.041	0.048	0.071
0.2	T	65.60	34.33	15.35	8.78	5.22	2.70
	Expected	20.25	12.57	7.55	5.42	3.89	2.36
	Monte Carlo p	0.019	0.020	0.035	0.060	0.071	0.118
0.5	T	33.75	18.23	8.72	5.33	3.38	1.86
	Expected	14.96	9.28	5.58	4.00	2.87	1.74
	Monte Carlo p	0.030	0.035	0.044	0.062	0.094	0.183
1	T	21.89	12.18	6.16	3.94	2.60	1.49
	Expected	12.26	7.61	4.57	3.28	2.36	1.43
	Monte Carlo p	0.030	0.032	0.057	0.061	0.104	0.204
2	T	14.84	8.52	4.55	3.03	2.07	1.21
	Expected	10.15	6.30	3.78	2.72	1.95	1.18
	Monte Carlo p	0.033	0.050	0.085	0.097	0.145	0.252
2	T	9.25	5.51	3.12	2.17	1.52	0.91
	Expected	7.72	4.79	2.88	2.07	1.48	0.899
	Monte Carlo p	0.101	0.109	0.133	0.192	0.218	0.266

Table 7.9 Jacquez's k-NN approach with Monte Carlo p-value with $N_{rep} = 999$ for 22 patients with Kaposi's sarcoma in the West Nile district of Uganda (data from McHardy *et al.*, 1984).

	k nearest neighbors									
	1	2	3	4	5	6	7	8	9	10
T	0.5	2.5	4.0	8.0	13.5	20.0	26.0	34.5	43.0	52.5
Expected	0.52	2.09	4.71	8.38	13.09	18.85	25.66	33.52	42.42	52.38
Monte Carlo p	0.575	0.396	0.678	0.582	0.419	0.334	0.431	0.320	0.378	0.438

the Knox test. As the study region $|A|$ covering all the data points, we used the polygonal study region shown in Figure 7.2, which approximates the boundary of the study region. To do this, we use the following R program:

R program for Figure 7.2

```
dat< − scan("McHardy.dat",list(x=0,y=0,t=0))
kap.pts< − as.points(dat$x,dat$y)
pointmap(kap.pts, xlim=c(230, 320), ylim=c(230, 400),
xlab=" Eastings ", ylab =" Northings " )
kap.poly< − spoints(scan("d:/book/kappoly.txt"))
polymap(Kap.poly, add=T)
```

Figure 7.3 shows two perspective plots of the surfaces (a) $\hat{D}(s,t)$ and (b) $\hat{D}_0(s,t)$. Especially, we can see in the perspective plot of $\hat{D}_0(s,t)$ that the excess risk suddenly increases at around time limit $t = 0$ and space limits $s = 2$ and 3, suggesting space-time interaction. These plots are produced using the following R program.

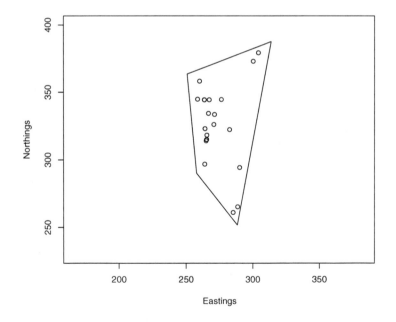

Fig. 7.2 Spatial locations of 22 cases of Kaposi's sarcoma in the West Nile district of Uganda.

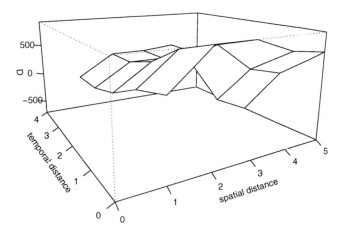

(a) $\hat{D}(s,t)$

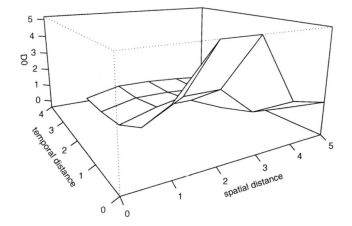

(b) $\hat{D}_0(s,t)$

Fig. 7.3 Perspective plots of the surface (a) $\hat{D}(s,t)$ and (b) $\hat{D}_0(s,t)$ for the spatial locations of 22 cases of Kaposi's sarcoma in the West Nile district of Uganda.

R program for Figure 7.3

```
kap1< − stkhat(kap.pts, dat$t, kap.poly, c(1955, 1980),seq(1,5),seq(0,
4))
g1< − matrix(kap1$ks)
g2< − matrix(kap1$kt)
g1g2< − g1 %*% t(g2)
turD< − kap1$kst − g1g2
persp(kap1$s, kap1$t, turD, theta = −30, phi = 15, expand = 0.5,
xlim=c(0,5), ylim=c(0,4), xlab="spatial distance",
ylab="temporal distance", zlab=" D ", ticktype = "detailed")
turD0< − kap1$kst / g1g2 − 1.0
persp(kap1$s, kap1$t, turD0, theta = −30, phi = 15, expand = 0.5,
xlim=c(0,5), ylim=c(0,4), xlab="spatial distance",
ylab="temporal distance", zlab=" D0 ", ticktype = "detailed")
```

Furthermore, in Figure 7.4, we show a scatter plot of $R(s,t)$ against $\hat{K}_1(s,t)\hat{K}_2(s,t)$ using the following R program:

R program for Figure 7.4

```
se< − stsecal(kap.pts,dat$t, kap.poly,c(1955, 1980),seq(1,5),seq(0,4))
Res< − turD / se
plot( g1g2, Res , ylim=c( −3, 6), xlab=" K1(s)K2(t) ",
ylab=" standardized residuals R(s,t) ")
abline(h=c(−2,2), lty=2)
```

Figure 7.4 also suggests the presence of space-time clustering derived from small temporal and spatial scales as seen on the surface of $\hat{D}_0(s,t)$. Finally, we performed two Monte Carlo tests with $N_{\text{rep}} = 999$ based on the Sum test statistic U_{sum} and the Max test statistic U_{max} using the R function **DiggleETAL.test** (Appendix).

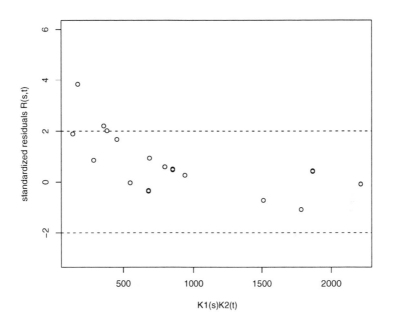

Fig. 7.4 Scatter plot of $R(s,t)$ against $\hat{K}_1(s,t)\hat{K}_2(s,t)$ for 22 cases of Kaposi's sarcoma in the West Nile district of Uganda.

Output from the R function DiggleETAL.test

```
>Nrep< − 999
>out< − DiggleETAL.test(kap.pts, dat$t, kap.poly, c(1955, 1980),
seq(1,5),seq(0, 4),Nrep)
>out$Sum.p.value
[1] 0.181
>out$Max.p.value
[1] 0.061
```

The observed Sum test statistic was $U_{\text{sum}} = 17.11$, and the Max test statistic was $D_{\text{max}} = 3.068$ at $s = 2,3$ and $t = 0$. The simulated p-value of the observed $U_{sum} = 17.11$ was $p = 0.181$ and that of the observed $U_{\text{max}} = 3.068$ was 0.061, which suggests mild evidence of space-time clustering. Histograms of simulated U_{sum} and U_{max} plus observed test statistics are shown in Figure 7.5.

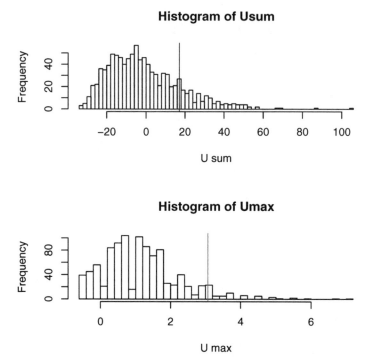

Fig. 7.5 Histograms of U_{sum} and U_{max} and locations of the observed U's.

7.6 Power Comparison

As described in the previous section, power comparisons have been performed by Chen, Mantel, and Klingberg (1984), Wartenberg and Greenberg (1990), and Jacquez (1996).

Euclidean distance vs. k-nearest neighbors

Especially, Jacquez (1996) described several deficiencies of the Knox and Mantel tests and several strengths of the k-NN test, and showed that the k-NN test has superior power relative to the Knox and Mantel tests in his simulation studies. However, any k-NN test fails to detect space-time clustering for the previous data on 22 patients with Kaposi's sarcoma without adjustment for multiple testing while Mantel's test detected significant clustering using Baker's adjustment for multiple testing. That is, the power of the test does depend on the unknown clustering process, and thus it will be quite difficult to determine the best method using simulated data. If the process of space-time clustering is related to a Euclidian metric rather than a nearest neighbors metric, then the test based on the former seems to be better and vice versa. Therefore, in real applications where we do not have enough information on the clustering process, both approaches should be applied.

Selection of Tests based on Euclidean distance

In general, Mantel's test based on a *clinal type* measure of closeness is more powerful than Knox's test based on a *hot-spot type* measure of closeness, as is shown in the example above. Diggle *et al.*'s K-function approach without edge correction is essentially equivalent to Knox's test statistic. Furthermore, to avoid multiple testing, Baker's Max test statistic (the same approach as Tango's Min P test statistic; for example, see (5.13), (6.20)) should be employed. Therefore, Baker's Max test for Mantel's test could be recommended as the first choice.

Adjustment for varying population growth rate

It has been known that tests for space-time interactions are biased when there are varying population growth rates in different regions. Therefore, when the difference in population growth rates is nonnegligible, Kulldorff and Hjalmars' Monte Carlo approach should be employed. In this case, we need to determine the population growth rate for each case with caution.

Chapter 8
Focused Tests for Spatial Clustering

Focused clustering studies examine raised disease risk around prespecified point sources such as nuclear installations and incinerators, which are illustrated by the following two examples.

Example 1

Table 8.1 shows the observed and expected numbers of infant deaths for each of ten zones from MSW incinerators "A" and "B", respectively. Do these data suggest any clustering of infant deaths around the incinerators?

Example 2

Figure 8.1 shows the residential locations of 57 cases (+) of larynx cancer and 917 controls (∘) and ten zones delimited by ten circles of radii of 1,2,...,10 km from a disused industrial incinerator in the Chorley-Ribble area of Lancashire, England.

Table 8.1 Observed and expected numbers of infant deaths for each of ten zones, $(j, j+1], j = 0, 1, ..., 9$ (km) from the municipal solid waste incinerator A in Japan.

	Zones										
	1	2	3	4	5	6	7	8	9	10	Total
Incinerator A											
Observed n_i	0	1	3	2	1	8	7	4	0	2	28
Expected e_i	0.041	0.701	1.128	1.634	1.868	5.738	4.550	3.617	3.792	4.931	28
O/E ratio	0.000	1.427	2.660	1.224	0.535	1.394	1.538	1.106	0.000	0.406	
Incinerator B											
Observed n_i	1	3	1	1	1	2	2	2	4	3	20
Expected e_i	0.998	0.724	1.611	1.623	1.270	1.116	1.820	1.377	3.709	5.752	20
O/E ratio	1.002	4.144	0.621	0.616	0.787	1.792	1.099	1.452	1.078	0.522	

T. Tango, *Statistical Methods for Disease Clustering*,
Statistics for Biology and Health, DOI 10.1007/978-1-4419-1572-6_8,
© Springer Science+Business Media, LLC 2010

Larynx cancer cases and controls

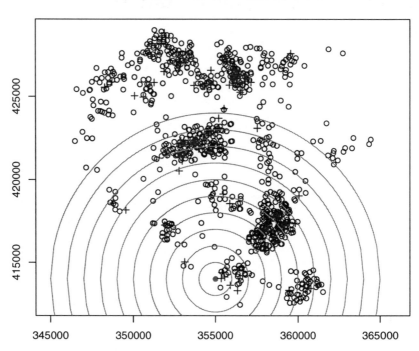

Fig. 8.1 Locations of larynx cancer cases (+) and controls (○) and ten zones delimited by ten circles of radii 1, 2,..., 10 km from a disused industrial incinerator in the Chorley-Ribble area of Lancashire, England. (This data set is from Splancs in R.)

(This data set is reproduced from Splancs in R.) Does this figure indicate a clustering of cancers around the now disused incinerator ?

8.1 Data

To test for clustering around the prespecified point source, we need to collect data on the location of the point source and each case for a defined geographic area during a specified study period. Throughout this chapter, it is assumed that

1. The total observed number of cases is n.
2. The study area is divided into m geographic regions (e.g., census tracts, counties, or states), where

a. The observed number of cases and the null expected number of cases of the disease under study in region i are denoted by n_i and e_i $(i = 1,...,m)$, respectively, with $n = n_1 + \cdots + n_m$.
b. The population size of region i is denoted by ξ_i.
c. The centroid of region i is denoted by (x_i, y_i).
d. The location of the point source is (x_0, y_0)
e. The distance between the ith region and the point source is defined as $d_i = \sqrt{(x_i - x_0)^2 + (y_i - y_0)^2}$.

8.2 Null Hypothesis vs. Alternative Hypothesis

A verbal expression of these two hypotheses taking childhood leukemia as an example will be

H_0 : There is no clustering of childhood leukemia around a nuclear
    reprocessing plant

H_1 : There is a clustering of childhood leukemia around a nuclear
    reprocessing plant

or we may say in terms of epidemiological investigation

H_0 : the risk of childhood leukemia is not increased near a nuclear
    reprocessing plant

H_1 : the risk of childhood leukemia is increased near a nuclear
    reprocessing plant

To define these hypotheses statistically, we shall consider the situation where we have regional count data unless otherwise noted. Let us consider the situation where an entire study area A is divided into m regions. The number of cases in the ith region is denoted by the random variable N_i with observed value n_i, $i = 1, 2, ..., m$. Under the null hypothesis H_0 of no clustering, the N_i are independent Poisson variables with mean e_i

$$H_0 : E(N_i) = e_i, \quad (i = 1,...,m) \tag{8.1}$$

where the e_i is the null expected number of cases of the ith region. The e_i is usually calculated using the rates r_k from some reference population and is called the *unconditional* null expected number of cases

$$e_i = \sum_{k=1}^{K} \xi_{ik} r_k, \quad (i = 1,...,m) \tag{8.2}$$

where ξ_{ik} denotes the number of individuals at risk or population size in the kth category of the set of potential confounders such as age and sex of the ith region.

However, there may often be situations in which the external rates r_k are considered inappropriate for some reason; for example, there might be a rural/urban effect related to the entire study area A. Then we will go on to take the conditional approach using the internally calculated rates r'_k

$$e_i = \sum_{k=1}^{K} \xi_{ik} r'_k = \sum_{k=1}^{K} \xi_{ik} \left(\frac{\sum_{j=1}^{m} n_{jk}}{\sum_{j=1}^{m} \xi_{jk}} \right), \quad (i = 1, ..., m) \tag{8.3}$$

where n_{jk} denotes the observed number of cases in the kth category of the set of potential confounders of the jth region. In the conditional approach, we have

$$\sum_{i=1}^{m} e_i = n \quad \text{(total observed number of cases)}$$

These e_i's are called *conditional* null expected numbers of cases. It should be recognized that standardizing internally would be hazardous in that the effect of the putative source of pollution could be reduced if, say, more elderly people live close to the source. It should be noted that focused tests based on the unconditional null expected number of cases are called *unconditional tests* and those based on the conditional null expected number of cases are called *conditional tests*. Then, an unconditional alternative hypothesis of clustering can be expressed as

$$H_1 : E(N_i) = \theta_i e_i, \quad N_i \sim \text{Poisson} \tag{8.4}$$

where the θ_i denote the region-specific relative risks. On the other hand, a conditional alternative hypothesis, given n, can be

$$H_1 : (N_1, ..., N_m) \sim \text{Multinomial distribution with probability } \boldsymbol{p} \tag{8.5}$$

where

$$\boldsymbol{p}' = (p_1, ..., p_m), \quad p_i = \frac{\theta_i e_i}{\sum_{j=1}^{m} \theta_j e_j} \tag{8.6}$$

In terms of the value of region-specific relative risks θ_i's, the null hypothesis will be

$$H_0 : \theta_1 = \theta_2 = \cdots = \theta_m \tag{8.7}$$

Regarding the alternative hypothesis, we can consider the *additive excess risk model*

$$\text{Excess risk hypothesis } H_1 : \quad \theta_i = 1 + g_i \varepsilon \quad (i = 1, ..., m) \tag{8.8}$$

as a natural alternative, where g_i denotes the exposure to the point source experienced by individuals in the ith region and is called the *exposure function* throughout this chapter. Generally, we do not have enough information on the exposure and then we have to replace g_i with a surrogate for the exposure; e.g., an inverse measure of distance to the point source. As another possibility, we may simply assume an order-restricted hypothesis or *decline in risk with distance from the prespecified point source*

$$\text{decline hypothesis } H_1 : \ \theta_{(1)} \geq \theta_{(2)} \geq \cdots \geq \theta_{(m)} \tag{8.9}$$

where $\theta_{(i)}$ denotes the relative risk for the region that is the ith nearest to the point source. However, the simple nonincreasing restriction (8.9) is not always valid. There may be a situation where the hazardous substance levels tend to have a peak at some distance from the putative source of the hazard. Therefore, an alternative for detecting a peak-decline trend is needed

$$\text{peak-decline hypothesis } H_1 : \ \theta_{(1)} \leq \cdots \leq \theta_{(l^*)} \geq \cdots \geq \theta_{(m)} \tag{8.10}$$

where the relative risk attains the peak at the region that is the l^*th nearest to the point source.

8.3 Historical Overview of Methods

(It should be noted that there are several other proposed methods not mentioned here. Furthermore, readers who are not interested in the history can skip this section.)

Since the 1980s there has been growing interest in the analysis of small-area data to investigate the relation between the risk of a disease and the proximity to a prespecified putative source of hazard. It is well-known that the apparent excess of cases of childhood leukemia near a nuclear reprocessing plant such as Seascale in the village of Sellafield has been extensively investigated (for example, see Bithell *et al.*, 1994). More recently, there has been great public concern about the health effects of so-called *dioxins*, organic compounds such as polychlorinated dibenzo-dioxins (PCDDs) and dibenzofurans (PCDFs) emitted from municipal solid waste incinerators (for example, see Elliott *et al.*, 1996).

The primary statistical problems arising in the traditional approach to these epidemiological studies are *post hoc* analyses of the *reported clusters* of cases near putative sources. Bias in the selection of regions due to prior knowledge of an apparent effect may cause multiple testing problems and subjectivity in interpreting the study results (Bithell and Stone, 1989; Bithell, 1992). To avoid these inferential problems, many statistical tests, called *focused tests*, to detect such an excess risk or a cluster of cases around a putative source have been proposed.

Stone's test (1988), among others, is very popular since it is based on traditional epidemiological estimates of the SMR or SIR (standardized mortality or incidence ratios). Stone (1988) proposed a nonparametric approach to testing the null hypothesis of no clustering against a monotone alternative H_1 (8.9). Stone considered a maximum likelihood ratio (MLR) test that, under the order-restricted H_1 (8.9), calculates the maximum likelihood estimators $\hat{\theta}_{(i)}$ and is easily obtained by using the so-called pool-adjacent violators algorithm (see Barlow *et al.*, 1972)

$$\hat{\theta}_{(i)} = \min_{s \leq i} \max_{t \geq i} \frac{\sum_{r=s}^{t} n_{(r)}}{\sum_{r=s}^{t} e_{(r)}} \quad i = 1, \ldots, m.$$

where $n_{(r)}$ and $e_{(r)}$ denote the observed and expected numbers of cases, respectively, for the region that is the rth nearest to the point source. Since there are order restrictions on the parameters, the usual asymptotic properties of the maximum likelihood ratio test are not guaranteed. Then, Stone (1988) proposed the first parameter estimator $\hat{\theta}_{(1)}$ under the order restriction as an alternative test statistic whose null distribution can be obtained without simulation. However, the power of the MLR test is generally higher than that based on $\hat{\theta}_{(1)}$ except for the case where nearly all the excess risk is concentrated very close to the putative source of the hazard. So, given the availability of cheap computer simulation, it may well be preferable to carry out a Monte Carlo test using the MLR test.

There are several applications of Stone's test. Elliot *et al.* (1992) apply Stone's test to examine the incidence of lung and laryngeal cancers around incinerators of waste solvents and oils at Charnock Richard in Lancashire (1972–1980), but could not reject the null hypothesis of no clustering. Elliot *et al.* (1996) extend this study to a cancer dataset in Great Britain in relation to solid waste incinerators and find some evidence for a decline in risk with distance from incinerators for several cancers. Dolk *et al.* (1997a) found the risk of adult leukemia during 1974–1986 to be elevated within 2 km of the Sutton Coldfield transmitter and a significant decline in risk with distance from the transmitter. Dolk *et al.* (1997b) extended their study to the vicinity of 20 high-power transmitters across Great Britain and found significant results. Michelozzi *et al.* (2002) examined the leukemia mortality among adults and childhood leukemia incidence within the 10 km area around the Vatican Radio high-power radio transmitter and found a significant decline in risk with increasing distance both for adult mortality and childhood leukemia incidence.

There are also several extensions of Stone's test. Morton-Jones, Diggle, and Elliot (1999) proposed an extension to allow for a region's specific covariate adjustment via a log-linear model

$$\log E(N_{(i)}) = \log\{e_{(i)} \theta_{(i)}\} + \sum_{j=1}^{p} x_{(i)j} \beta_j$$

where the x_{ij}'s are the values of each of p explanatory variables in each of n regions and the β_j's are unknown regression parameters. Their methods are illustrated with data on the incidence of stomach cancer near two municipal incinerators. Diggle, Morris, and Morton-Jones (1999) developed Stone's approach for case-control data consisting of the locations of individual cases and controls. They also considered the covariate adjustment. They illustrate their methods with two kinds of data; data on larynx cancers and lung cancers near a now disused industrial incinerator and data on asthma in children in relation to the distance of their residence from the nearest main road.

Stone's test, however, has been shown to be not so powerful in the literature. If we have enough information on the region-specific relative risk of the alternative hypothesis H_1 given in (8.4), then the most powerful test can be of the form (Bithell, 1995)

$$T = \sum_{i=1}^{m} n_i \log(\theta_i) \geq t_0$$

where t_0 should be chosen to ensure the correct type I error α for the test. However, it is very rare that we have enough information on θ_i's. Bithell called this kind of test a linear risk score (LRS) test using θ_i as scores. When we are interested in detecting the clusters of rare diseases under study around the prespecified putative point source and we cannot assume values for the relative risks θ_i, an alternative is to consider a simple ordering (8.9). Bithell then examines LRS tests by replacing the unknown $\theta_{(i)}$ by a suitable relative risk function of distance such as "1/distance" and the reciprocal of distance rank. Of course, there are many other possibilities for monotonic functions of distance. Bithell et al. (1994) compared the power of LRS tests with several relative risk functions with Stone's MLR tests and found that LRS tests are more powerful than Stone's tests. Bithell et al. (1994) applied LRS tests to data from childhood leukemia incidence around 23 nuclear installations in England and Wales where significant results are obtained at only two sites, Sellafield and Burghfield.

As a locally most powerful test, on the other hand, score tests have been proposed as an alternative test (Waller et al., 1992; Lawson, 1993; Tango, 1995). Under the additive excess risk model (8.8), the null hypothesis and the alternative hypothesis can be defined as

$$H_0 : \varepsilon = 0, \quad H_1 : \varepsilon > 0$$

Therefore, the efficient score statistic is

$$U = \sum_{i=1}^{m} g_i(n_i - e_i)$$

which is asymptotically normally distributed with mean 0 and variance equal to the inverse of the Fisher Information

$$\text{Var}(U) = \left\{ \sum_{i=1}^{m} e_i g_i^2 - \left(\sum_{i=1}^{m} e_i g_i \right)^2 / n \right\}$$

where g_i is a function that relates *inversely* to geographic distance d_i from the point source. If the e_i is unconditionally calculated, then it should be replaced by $n e_i / \sum_{j=1}^{m} e_j$. It should be noted that the most powerful test for this alternative is the LRS test based on $\sum_{i=1}^{m} n_i \log(1 + g_i \varepsilon)$, which is asymptotically (as $\varepsilon \to 0$) equivalent to the efficient score test based on $\sum_{i=1}^{m} n_i g_i$, the latter having the advantage that it does not depend on the unknown ε.

Simulation studies in Waller and Lawson (1995) and Waller (1996) show that the score test based on inverse distance has greater power than Stone's test based on $\theta_{(1)}$ and other tests against alternatives that they thought were of more practical interest. However, like the score or the relative risk functions required in the LRS tests, the choice of transformation we use to achieve a suitable *inverse measure* of distance introduces an element of arbitrariness and will cause multiple testing problems. It should be noted here that these tests are identical in form to score tests used in epidemiologic settings where one knows exposure values for each of several strata (Breslow and Day, 1987). Waller *et al.* (1992) illustrate the score tests with leukemia incidence data in upstate New York (1978–1982), with inactive hazardous waste sites as point sources. In a study to examine the bronchitis mortality around a chemical reprocessing plant in Bonnybridge, central Scotland (1980–1982), Lawson (1993) illustrates the score tests. Michelozzi *et al.* (2002) apply the score tests to examine the leukemia mortality among adults and childhood leukemia incidence within the 10 km area around the Vatican Radio high-power radio transmitter. They consider five different functions for g_i, and two functions give a significant decline in risk with increasing distance for childhood leukemia incidence, leading to a problem of multiple testing. When there are several foci to be specified simultaneously, Tango (1995) proposed a generalized score statistic.

In a way similar to Morton-Jones, Diggle, and Elliot (1999), we can easily consider an extension of the score test that allows for adjustment of region-specific covariates via a log-linear model

$$\log E(N_i) = \log\{e_i(1 + g_i \varepsilon)\} + \sum_{j=1}^{p} x_{ij} \beta_j$$

Tango (2002) proposed extensions of score tests that (1) allow us to select the best prespecified parametric exposure functions to avoid multiple testing problems and (2) can be applied to a possible situation where the hazardous substance levels have a peak at some distance from a point source. For the decline hypothesis (8.9), Tango (2002) considered the double exponential decay function of exposure $g_i(\lambda)$ with one parameter λ

$$g_i(\lambda) = \exp\left\{-4\left(\frac{d_i}{\lambda}\right)^2\right\}$$

where λ is the scale parameter of the mode of the cluster and $g_i(\lambda)$ attains nearly zero at $d_{ij} = \lambda$. This decay function has been used in Tango's (1995, 2000) spatial clustering index as a measure of closeness between two regions. Large λ will give a test sensitive to a large cluster and small λ sensitive to a small cluster. To take the multiple testing problem associated with the selection of λ into account, Tango (2002) proposed, as an extended score test, *the minimum of the profile p-value of U for λ*, where λ varies continuously from a small value near zero upward to a large value given by users. For the purpose of detecting a peak-decline trend, Lawson (1993, p.372) proposed a score test based on the model

$$\theta_i = \exp(\beta_0 \log(d_i) + \beta_1 d_i)$$

Although this function of distance can surely express some peak-decline curves for some parameter values, the score test derived under this model cannot be an appropriate test for peak-decline trend since this model also assumes the exposure is proportional to the distance. Tango (2002) proposed the test statistic P_{decline} for detecting a decline trend

$$P_{\text{decline}} = \min_{\lambda} \Pr\{U_\lambda > u_\lambda \mid H_0, \lambda\} = 1 - \Phi\left(\max_{\lambda} \frac{u_\lambda}{\sqrt{\text{Var}(U_\lambda)}}\right)$$

where u_λ is the observed test statistic as a function of λ, and $\Phi()$ denotes the standard normal distribution function. A practical implementation of this procedure is to use "line search" by discretizing λ. The null distribution of P_{decline} can be obtained by Monte Carlo testing. Obviously, the test statistic P_{decline} above is equivalent to the simpler Max test statistic:

$$T_{\text{decline}} = \max_{\lambda} \frac{U_\lambda}{\sqrt{\text{Var}(U_\lambda)}}$$

To make the procedure above applicable to the peak-decline hypothesis (8.10), Tango (2002) modified the exposure decay function as

$$g_i = \begin{cases} g^{(0)}(d_i, s) \geq 1 & \text{if } d_i < s \ (s > 0) \\ g^{(1)}(d_i, s) \leq 1, & \text{otherwise} \end{cases}$$

where $g^{(0)}(s,s) = g^{(1)}(s,s) = 1$ and the g_i is defined as a monotone exposure function when $s = 0$. Here also, the choice of these functions may be variable depending on the situation, but here, for ease of interpretation, Tango chooses the particular functions

$$g^{(0)}(d,s) = 1 - 4\frac{a-1}{s^2}d(d-s)$$

$$g^{(1)}(d,s) = \exp\left\{-4\left(\frac{d-s}{\lambda}\right)^2\right\}$$

where $g^{(0)}$ attains a predetermined constant a at distance $d = s/2$. The choice of a also looks arbitrary, but we have only to set a larger than a possible maximum relative risk, say $a = 2.0$ or 3.0. In our experience, the result does not change essentially by choosing a greater than the maximum relative risk. However, in terms of estimation, the function above seems to be a little unrealistic in that the first partial derivative with respect to d is not continuous. Then the extended score test devised for a peak-decline trend including the decline trend is given by

$$T_{\text{peak-decline}} = \max_{\lambda,s} \frac{U_{\lambda,s}}{\sqrt{\text{Var}(U_{\lambda,s})}}$$

A practical implementation of this procedure is also to use a "numerical search" by discretizing λ and s. The null distribution of $T_{\text{peak-decline}}$ can be obtained by Monte Carlo testing. Needless to say, whether T_{decline} or $T_{\text{peak-decline}}$ should be used depends strongly on prior knowledge of exposures and also the availability of detailed address information of cases and controls around the point sources. In general, a monotone declining trend is a good approximation for an epidemiological study based on centroids of small areas.

Tango et al. (2004) used Stone's unconditional test and Tango's conditional score tests to examine the adverse reproductive outcomes associated with maternal residential proximity (within 10 km) to 63 municipal solid waste incinerators with high dioxin emission levels in Japan in 1997–1998. Regarding Tango's conditional score test result, p-values from each municipal solid waste incinerator are combined using a meta-analysis based on the weighted inverse normal method (Hedges and Olkin, 1985). As a result, (1) all of Stone's unconditional tests for decline in risk with distance were not statistically significant, (2) all the conditional tests for the decline hypothesis were not significant, and (3), however, a significant peak-decline in risk with distance was found for infant deaths and infant deaths with all congenital malformations combined, where a "peak" is detected around 1–2 km for some incinerators.

Kulldorff's spatial scan statistic, already described in Chapters 5 and 6, can be used for detecting clusters around the prespecified point source by considering only the circles with the centroid of the prespecified point source. For example, Viel et al. (2000) examined the spatial distribution of soft-tissue sarcomas and non-Hodgkin's lymphomas around a French municipal solid waste incinerator with high emission levels of dioxin using SaTScan. The highly significant most likely clusters found were identical for soft-tissue sarcomas and non-Hodgkin's lymphomas and included two adjacent electoral wards around the municipal solid waste incinerator. However, Kulldorff's spatial scan statistic tests the null hypothesis H_0 against the alternative hypothesis of a *hot-spot* cluster

$$\text{hot-spot hypothesis } H_1 : \theta_{(1)} = \cdots = \theta_{(k)} > \theta_{(k+1)} = \cdots = \theta_{(m)} \qquad (8.11)$$

where the $(k-1)$ nearest neighbors to the point source, $\{(1),..., (k)\}$, that attains the maximum likelihood is defined as the most likely cluster (MLC). Therefore, it is expected to be less powerful against the alternatives *decline hypothesis* and *peak-decline hypothesis*.

Besag and Newell's test (1991) introduced in Section 5.3 can be used as a focused test for spatial clustering. However, as in the case of general tests for spatial clustering, it is quite difficult for users to determine the appropriate cluster size k a *priori*, and thus this test clearly faces multiple testing problems by repeating the test with a number of plausible values of k.

Diggle (1990) develops a methodology for fitting a class of inhomogeneous Poisson point process models using a nonparametric kernel smoothing approach to describe raised incidence near a prespecified point source. Diggle and Rowlingson (1994) develop a conditional approach to inference that converts the point process model to a nonlinear binary regression model for the spatial variation in risk, which is shown to be more reliable than Diggle's (1990) original point process setting.

Regarding review papers on the detection of clustering around putative point sources, see, for example, Hills and Alexander (1989), Muirhead and Darby (1989), Marshall (1991), Elliott, Martuzzi, and Shaddick (1995) and Lawson and Waller (1996).

8.4 Selected Methods

We consider here only the *conditional tests* since the selection of an appropriate external rate is not so easy and so the calculated expected number of cases may not be trustworthy in an absolute sense in practice.

8.4.1 Stone's Test

Goal: To calculate the maximum likelihood ratio test statistic and evaluate its significance. A significantly large value would indicate evidence of spatial clustering around the prespecified point source of the disease under study; i.e., *there is a significant decline in risk with increasing distance from the prespecified point source*.
Null hypothesis H_0: (8.7)
Alternative hypothesis H_1: (8.9)

Test statistic

The test statistic is the maximum likelihood ratio (MLR) test statistic

$$T_S = 2 \sum_{i=1}^{m} n_i \left\{ \log \hat{\theta}_{(i)} - \log \left(\frac{\sum_{j=1}^{m} \hat{\theta}_{(i)} e_{(i)}}{\sum_{j=1}^{m} e_{(j)}} \right) \right\} \tag{8.12}$$

where $\hat{\theta}_{(i)}$'s are maximum likelihood estimators, which are easily obtained by using the so-called pool-adjacent violators algorithm (see Barlow *et al.*, 1972)

$$\hat{\theta}_{(i)} = \min_{s \leq i} \max_{t \geq i} \frac{\sum_{r=s}^{t} n_{(r)}}{\sum_{r=s}^{t} e_{(r)}}, \quad i = 1, ..., m. \tag{8.13}$$

where $n_{(r)}$ and $e_{(r)}$ denote the observed and expected numbers of cases, respectively, for the region that is the rth nearest to the point source.

Null distribution

Monte Carlo hypothesis testing is required to obtain the null distribution of T_S and the Monte Carlo simulated p-value (2.17).

8.4.2 Bithell's Linear Risk Score Test

Goal: To calculate the linear rank score test statistic and evaluate its significance. A significantly large value would indicate evidence of spatial clustering around the prespecified point source of the disease under study; i.e., *there is a significant decline in risk with increasing distance from the prespecified point source.*
Null hypothesis H_0: (8.7)
Alternative hypothesis H_1: (8.9)

Test statistic

The test statistic is the most powerful test when the relative risk θ_i is known:

$$T_B = \sum_{i=1}^{m} n_i \log(\theta_i) \tag{8.14}$$

where the θ_i's are user defined scores. Bithell *et al.* (1994) and Bithell (1995) called this test statistic "linear risk score (LRS) test" and considered several score θ_i's such as $\theta_i = 1/d_i$, $1/(1+d_i)$, $1/(1+d_i)^2$, and the reciprocal of distance rank.

Null distribution

Monte Carlo hypothesis testing is required to obtain the null distribution of T_S and the Monte Carlo simulated p-value (2.17).

8.4.3 Waller and Lawson's Score Test

Goal: To calculate the efficient score test statistic and evaluate its significance. A significantly large value would indicate evidence of spatial clustering around the prespecified point source of the disease under study; i.e., *there is a significant decline in risk with increasing distance from the prespecified point source.*

Null hypothesis H_0: (8.7)
Alternative hypothesis H_1: (8.9)

Test statistic

The test statistic is based upon the efficient score for the additive excess risk model (8.8)

$$T_{WL} = \frac{\sum_{i=1}^{m} g_i(n_i - e_i)}{\sqrt{\sum_{i=1}^{m} e_i g_i^2 - (\sum_{i=1}^{m} e_i g_i)^2 / n}} \tag{8.15}$$

where the exposure function g_i is a user-defined function such as $g_i = 1/d_i$, $1/(1 + d_i)$, $1/(1 + d_i)^2$, and the reciprocal of distance rank.

Null distribution

The null distribution of the test statistic T_{WL} is asymptotically normally distributed with mean 0 and variance 1. However, for a small sample size n, Monte Carlo hypothesis testing is required to obtain the null distribution of T_S and the Monte Carlo simulated p-value (2.17).

8.4.4 Tango's Score Test for Decline Trend

Goal: To calculate the maximum of the efficient score test statistic over the value λ of the exposure function within the user-defined range $[\lambda_L, \lambda_U]$ and evaluate its significance. A significantly large value would indicate evidence of spatial clustering around the prespecified point source of the disease under study; i.e., *there is a significant decline in risk with increasing distance from the prespecified point source*.
Null hypothesis H_0: (8.7)
Alternative hypothesis H_1: (8.9)

Test statistic

The test statistic is the Max test statistic T_{decline},

$$T_{\text{decline}} = \max_{\lambda_L \le \lambda \le \lambda_u} \frac{\sum_{i=1}^{m} g_i(\lambda)(n_i - e_i)}{\sqrt{\sum_{i=1}^{m} e_i g_i(\lambda)^2 - (\sum_{i=1}^{m} e_i g_i(\lambda))^2 / n}} = T_{WL}(\lambda^*)$$

$$\tag{8.16}$$

where

$$g_i(\lambda) = \exp\left\{-4\left(\frac{d_i}{\lambda}\right)^2\right\} \tag{8.17}$$

and λ^* attains the maximum of T_{decline}.

Null distribution

Monte Carlo hypothesis testing is required to obtain the null distribution of T_{decline} and the Monte Carlo simulated p-value (2.17).

8.4.5 Tango's Score Test for Peak-Decline Trend

Goal: To calculate the maximum of the efficient score test statistic over the values λ and s of the exposure function within the user-defined ranges $[\lambda_L, \lambda_U]$ and $[s_L, s_U]$, respectively, and evaluate its significance. A significantly large value would indicate evidence of spatial clustering around the prespecified point source of the disease under study; i.e., *there is a significant peak-decline trend in risk with increasing distance from the prespecified point source.*
Null hypothesis H_0: (8.7)
Alternative hypothesis H_1: (8.10)

Test statistic

The test statistic is

$$T_{\text{peak-decline}} = \max_{\lambda_L \leq \lambda \leq \lambda_u,\, s_L \leq s \leq s_u} \frac{\sum_{i=1}^m g_i(\lambda,s)(n_i - e_i)}{\sqrt{\sum_{i=1}^m e_i g_i(\lambda,s)^2 - \left(\sum_{i=1}^m e_i g_i(\lambda,s)\right)^2 / n}}$$
$$= T_{WL}(\lambda^*, s^*) \tag{8.18}$$

where $[\lambda_L, \lambda_u]$ and $[s_L, s_U]$ are the user-specified ranges and

$$g_i(\lambda,s) = \begin{cases} 1 - 4\frac{a-1}{s^2}d(d-s), & \text{if } d_i \leq s \ (s \geq 0) \\ \exp\{-4(\frac{d-s}{\lambda})^2\}, & \text{otherwise} \end{cases} \tag{8.19}$$

where $g_i(\lambda,s)$ attains a predetermined peak a at distance $d = s/2$. The choice of a also looks arbitrary, but we have only to set a larger than a possible maximum relative risk, say $a = 2.0$ or 3.0. It should be noted that the test statistic for the peak-decline model includes that for the decline model in that it is equivalent to the test statistic for the decline trend when $s = 0$.

Null distribution

Monte Carlo hypothesis testing is required to obtain the null distribution of $T_{\text{peak-decline}}$ and the Monte Carlo simulated p-value (2.17).

8.4.6 Diggle, Morris, and Morton-Jones' Test Based on Case-Control Point Data

Goal: To calculate the maximum likelihood ratio test statistic and evaluate its significance. A significantly large value would indicate evidence of spatial clustering around the prespecified point source of the disease under study; i.e., *there is a significant decline in risk with increasing distance from the prespecified point source.*

Data

The notation defined in Section 8.1 cannot be applied here because we are concerned with case-control point data and we need new definitions. Let (x_i, y_i), $i = 1, ..., n_0$ denote the locations of n cases of a disease under study and (x_i, y_i), $i = n_0 + 1, ..., n_0 + n_1$ denote the locations of m controls, defined to be a random sample from the population at risk. Let (x_0, y_0) denote the location of the pre-specified point source. Then the distance between the ith location and the point source is $d_i = \sqrt{(x_i - x_0)^2 + (y_i - y_0)^2}$.

Null hypothesis and alternative hypothesis

$$H_0 : \text{ the risk of disease is independent of spatial location} \tag{8.20}$$

$$H_1 : \text{ the risk of disease is a nonincreasing function of the distance}$$

$$\text{from a prespecified point source} \tag{8.21}$$

Let $Y_i, i = 1, ..., n_0 + n_1$ denote indicator random variables that take the value 1 if the corresponding individual i is a case and 0 if i is a control. Then, conditional on the $n_0 + n_1$ locations, the indicator variables Y_i are mutually independent Bernoulli random variables under H_0. In other words, the null hypothesis of no clustering can be stated as

$$H_0 : \text{ the observed } n_0 \text{ case series is a random sample from the entire}$$

$$\text{sample of size } n_0 + n_1 \text{ combining cases and controls} \tag{8.22}$$

The null hypothesis (8.22) is called a *random labeling hypothesis*, in which we can make a permutational inference conditional on the observed locations of cases and controls. Further, let $\theta_i = \Pr\{Y_i = 1\}$. Then, the two hypotheses above are

$$H_0 : \quad \theta_{(1)} = \theta_{(2)} = \cdots = \theta_{(n_0+n_1)} \tag{8.23}$$

$$H_1 : \quad \theta_{(1)} \geq \theta_{(2)} \geq \cdots \geq \theta_{(n_0+n_1)} \tag{8.24}$$

where $\theta_{(i)}$ denotes the relative risk for the region that is the ith nearest to the point source. Under H_1, the maximum likelihood estimators of the θ_i are easily obtained by the pool-adjacent violators algorithm.

Test statistic

The test statistic is the maximum likelihood ratio (MLR) test statistic

$$T_D = 2 \sum_{i=1}^{n_0+n_1} \left\{ y_{(i)} \log \frac{\hat{\theta}_{(i)}}{\bar{\theta}} + (1 - y_{(i)}) \log \frac{1 - \hat{\theta}_{(i)}}{1 - \bar{\theta}} \right\} \qquad (8.25)$$

where $\bar{\theta} = n_0/(n_0 + n_1)$ and the $\hat{\theta}_{(i)}$'s are maximum likelihood estimators under H_1 given by

$$\hat{\theta}_{(i)} = \min_{s \leq i} \max_{t \geq i} \frac{\sum_{r=s}^{t} y_{(r)}}{t - s + 1}, \quad i = 1, \dots, n_0 + n_1 \qquad (8.26)$$

Null distribution

Monte Carlo hypothesis testing is required under the random labeling hypothesis to obtain the null distribution of T_D and the Monte Carlo simulated p-value (2.17).

8.5 Illustration with Real Data

In this section, some selected methods will be illustrated with three types of published data: (1) infant deaths around municipal solid waste incinerators (Tango *et al.*, 2004); (2) leukemia cases near inactive hazardous waste sites (Waller *et al.*, 1992, 1994); and (3) larynx and lung cancers near a disused incinerator (Diggle, 1990; Diggle and Rowlinson, 1994; Diggle, Morris, and Morton-Jones, 1999).

8.5.1 Infant Deaths Around Municipal Solid Waste Incinerators

Tango *et al.* (2004) examine the association of adverse reproductive outcomes with mothers living within 10 km from 63 municipal solid waste (MSW) incinerators with high dioxin emission levels (above 80 ng international toxic equivalents TEQ/m3) during 1997–1998 in Japan. The selected reproductive outcomes studied were female live births (male/female sex ratio at birth), low birthweight (weighing less than 2500 g), very low birthweight (weighing less than 1500 g), infant deaths (under one year), infant deaths with congenital malformations, neonatal deaths (under four weeks), neonatal deaths with congenital malformations, early neonatal deaths (under one week), early neonatal deaths with congenital malformations, spontaneous fetal deaths (noninduced deaths before the complete expulsion or extraction from the mother after the 12th week of gestation), and spontaneous fetal deaths with congenital malformations.

Each study area was divided into ten subareas (called "zones") delimited by ten circles of radii 1, 2,..., 10 km. The statistical analysis of the association between maternal proximity to MSW incinerators and adverse reproductive outcome was primarily based upon the observed (O) and expected (E) numbers of cases. The expected number of cases was calculated using national rates on all live births, fetal deaths, and infant deaths that occurred during 1997–1998 in Japan, where national rates were stratified by potential confounding factors available from the corresponding vital statistics records: maternal age, gestational age, birthweight, total previous deliveries, past experience of fetal deaths, and type of paternal occupation. This procedure is very similar to that described in detail by Shaddick and Elliott (1996). As formal tests, Tango used Stone's unconditional test and Tango's conditional test for decline in risk (O/E ratio) with distance from the incinerator. Motivated by the dioxin levels in soils measured in the vicinity of MSW incinerators where a peak of concentration was found around 2 km from the incinerator, Tango *et al.* (2004) also applied Tango's conditional test for "peak-decline" in risk with distance, where the location of "peak" was restricted to be one of three zones, 0–1 km (decline model), 1–2 km, and 2–3 km.

To illustrate the selected methods with real data, we select two typical MSW incinerators, A and B, from 63 MSW incinerators, and we show observed and expected numbers of infant deaths for each of ten zones from MSW incinerators "A" and "B" in Table 8.1. The trend of risk of infant death around the MSW incinerator A seems to be an example of "decline in risk with distance from the point source" and that of risk of infant death around the MSW incinerator B seems to be an example of peak-decline in risk with distance with peak 1–2 km. In this special application, we considered the distance between the jth zone and the MSW incinerator to be defined as $d_j =| j |$.

8.5.1.1 Infant Deaths Around MSW Incinerator A

Stone's MLR test

First, we shall apply Stone's MLR test where the null distribution is obtained by Monte Carlo hypothesis testing with $N_{rep} = 9999$. Output from the R function **Stone.test** (Appendix) for Stone's MLR test with a Monte Carlo simulated p-value is shown below.

Output from the R function Stone.test

```
> Nrep< - 9999
> ob< - c(0, 1, 3, 2, 1, 8, 7, 4, 0, 2)
> ex< - c(0.041,0.701,1.128,1.634,1.868,5.738,4.550,3.617,3.792,4.931)
> out< - Stone.test(ob,ex,Nrep)
> out$Test.statistic
[1] 5.294094
> signif(out$Estimate,4)
[1] 2.139 2.139 2.139 1.305 1.305 1.305 1.305 1.106 0.229 0.229
> out$p.value
[1] 0.0104
```

The observed test statistic is $T_S = 5.294$ with simulated p-value $p = 0.0104$. The maximum likelihood estimates $\hat{\theta}_{(i)}$ are 2.139, 2.139, 2.139, 1.305, 1.305, 1.305, 1.305, 1.106, 0.229, 0.229.

Bithell's linear risk score test

Second, we shall apply Bithell's LRS test where the null distribution is obtained by Monte Carlo hypothesis testing with $N_{rep} = 9999$. Output from the R function **Bithell.test** (Appendix) for Bithell's LRS test with an exposure function $g_i = 1/d_i$ is shown below.

Output from the R function Bithell.test

```
> Nrep< - 9999
> d< - 1:10
> g< - 1/d
> out< - Bithell.test(ob,ex,g,Nrep)
> out$Test.statistic
[1] -49.24939
> out$p.value
[1] 0.0258
```

The observed test statistic is $T_B = -49.25$ with simulated p-value $p = 0.0258$. In order to examine the impact of the exposure function g_i on the test result, we shall repeat Bithell's LRS test by changing exposure functions $g_i = 1/d_i^a$, $a = 0.2, 0.5, 1, 2, 3$. All the p-values are the same as that of $a = 1$, indicating that Bithell's

LRS test is not so sensitive to the selection of g_i.

Waller and Lawson's score test

Third, we shall apply the Waller and Lawson's score test with the exposure function $g_i = 1/d_i$ where the null distribution is obtained by Monte Carlo hypothesis testing with $N_{rep} = 9999$. Output from the R function **WallerLawson.test** (Appendix) for the Waller-Lawson score test with Monte Carlo simulated p-value is shown below.

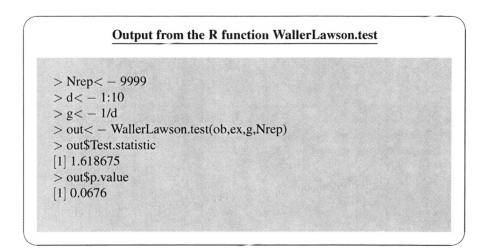

Output from the R function WallerLawson.test

```
> Nrep< − 9999
> d< − 1:10
> g< − 1/d
> out< − WallerLawson.test(ob,ex,g,Nrep)
> out$Test.statistic
[1] 1.618675
> out$p.value
[1] 0.0676
```

The observed test statistic is $T_{WL} = 1.619$ with simulated p-value $p = 0.0676$. In order to examine the impact of the exposure function g_i on the test result, we shall repeat Waller and Lawson's score test by changing the exposure functions $g_i = 1/d_i^a$, $a = 0.2, 0.5, 1, 2, 3$. Their results are $p = 0.0277, 0.0429, 0.0676, 0.13098$, and 0.1867, respectively, indicating that as the value of a increases, the p-value also tends to increase. That is, the score test is quite sensitive to the selection of g_i.

Tango's score test for decline trend

Fourth, we shall apply Tango's score test for the decline trend where the null distribution is obtained by Monte Carlo hypothesis testing with $N_{rep} = 9999$. We shall evaluate the maximum over the values of $\lambda \in \{2, 4, ..., 40\}$. Output from the R function **TangoF.test** (Appendix) for Tango's score test for the decline trend with Monte Carlo simulated p-value is shown below.

Output from the R function TangoF.test

```
> Nrep< −b9999
> d< − 1:10
> lam< − 2*(1:20)
> out< − TangoF.test(ob,ex,d,lam,Nrep)
> signif(out$Test.statistics,4)
0.2838 1.1880 1.5310 1.8410 2.0820 2.2220 2.2980 2.3420 2.3680
2.3840 2.3950 2.4020 2.4080 2.4120 2.4150 2.4170 2.4190 2.4210
2.4220 2.4230
> out$Max.statistic
[1] 2.423075
> out$p.value
[1] 0.0453
```

The observed test statistic is $T_{decline} = 2.423$ with simulated p-value $p = 0.0453$. **Test.statistics** which denotes the test statistics $T_{WL}(\lambda)$, $\lambda = 2, 4, ..., 40$ indicates that the maximum attains at $\lambda^* = 40$.

5. Tango's score test for peak-decline trend

Fifth, we shall apply Tango's score test for the peak-decline trend where the null distribution is obtained by Monte Carlo hypothesis testing with $N_{rep} = 9999$. To obtain $T_{peak\text{-}decline}$ defined in (8.18), we shall conduct a two-dimensional search over the grids (λ, s) defined by combinations of discrete values of $\lambda \in \{2, 4, ..., 40\}$ and $s \in \{0, 1, 2, 3, 4\}$. The range of s is determined according to some observed peak-decline decay curves of exposure levels experienced in a few investigations regarding atmospheric levels of pollutants such as polychlorinated dibenzodioxins (PCDDs) and dibenzofurans (PCDFs) around waste incinerators. Output from the R function **TangoFPD.test** (Appendix) for Tango's score test for the peak-decline trend with Monte Carlo simulated p-value is shown below.

Output from the R function TangoFPD.test

```
> Nrep< − 9999
> d< − 1:10
> lam< − 2*(1:20)
> s< − c(0,1,2,3,4)
> out< − TangoFPD.test(ob,ex,d,lam,s,Nrep)
> out$Test.statistics
[1,] 1.037094 1.3024155 1.545655 1.508090 1.797020
[2,] 1.503923 1.2905791 1.815365 2.113742 2.173718
[3,] 1.710983 1.6086651 2.236524 2.395693 2.137911
[4,] 2.015623 1.8719238 2.434335 2.443770 1.993471
[5,] 2.208765 1.9722316 2.496131 2.408170 1.837922
[6,] 2.307024 1.9756255 2.495787 2.341154 1.698458
[7,] 2.357305 1.9274712 2.463258 2.263916 1.582573
[8,] 2.384697 1.8503353 2.413198 2.187406 1.489501
[9,] 2.400678 1.7570166 2.354831 2.117033 1.415631
[10,] 2.410595 1.6560787 2.294311 2.054853 1.357007
[11,] 2.417083 1.5536254 2.235494 2.001080 1.310209
[12,] 2.421519 1.4538850 2.180522 1.955068 1.272529
[13,] 2.424670 1.3595500 2.130370 1.915856 1.241892
[14,] 2.426979 1.2721100 2.085289 1.882444 1.216735
[15,] 2.428718 1.1921816 2.045116 1.853910 1.195877
[16,] 2.430058 1.1197985 2.009488 1.829456 1.178423
[17,] 2.431113 1.0546384 1.977954 1.808408 1.163693
[18,] 2.431956 0.9961852 1.950050 1.790208 1.151161
[19,] 2.432642 0.9438378 1.925337 1.774393 1.140419
[20,] 2.433207 0.8969776 1.903410 1.760587 1.131149
> out$Max.statistic
[1] 2.496131
> out$p.value
[1] 0.0557
```

The observed test statistic is $T_{\text{peak-decline}} = 2.496$ with simulated p-value $p = 0.0557$. **Test.statistics**, whose values are $T_{WL}(\lambda, s)$, $\lambda = 2, 4, ..., 40$, $s = 0, 1, ..., 4$, indicate that the maximum is attained at $\lambda^* = 40$ and $s^* = 0$; i.e., the pattern of risk is a "decline in risk with distance".

Kulldorff's spatial scan statistic

For reference, let us apply Kulldorff's spatial scan statistic using SaTScan with $N_{\text{rep}} = 9999$. To do a focused test with SaTScan, we have only to use **Grid File** with only a single grid point reflecting the coordinates of the point source. The

Table 8.2 Observed and expected numbers of infant deaths for each of ten zones $(j, j+1], j =$ $0, 1, ..., 9$ km from the municipal solid waste incinerator A in Japan. Also shown are the O/E ratio, Stone's MLE, and estimated p-values based on Monte Carlo testing with 9999 replications for three tests.

	Zones										
	1	2	3	4	5	6	7	8	9	10	Total
Observed n_i	0	1	3	2	1	8	7	4	0	2	28
Expected e_i	0.041	0.701	1.128	1.634	1.868	5.738	4.550	3.617	3.792	4.931	28
O/E ratio		0.000	1.427	2.660	1.224	0.535	1.394	1.538	1.106	0.000	0.406
Stone's MLE	2.139	2.139	2.139	1.305	1.305	1.305	1.305	1.106	0.229	0.229	

Stone's MLR test: $p = 0.0104$.
Bithell's LRS test with $g_i = 1/d_i$: $p = 0.0258$.
Waller and Lawson's score test with $g_i = 1/d_i$: $p = 0.0676$.
Tango's score test for decline trend: $p = 0.0453$ ($\lambda^* = 40$).
Tango's score test for peak-decline trend: $p = 0.0557$ ($s^* = 0, \lambda^* = 40$).

identified MLC is composed of five nearest neighbors to the point source (0–6 km zone), and the p-value is 0.1758. As expected, the resultant p-value is the largest among the six tests applied.

7. Summary of the results

The results above are shown in Table 8.2. In this data set, a significant clustering at the 5% level around the MSW incinerator A was detected by Stone's MLR test ($p = 0.0104$), Bithell's LRS test with $g = 1/d$ ($p = 0.0258$), and Tango's score test for decline trend ($p = 0.0453$). Although Waller and Lawson's score test with $g = 1/d$ ($p = 0.0676$) and Tango's score test for peak-decline trend ($p = 0.0557$) cannot detect significant clustering, the differences in p-values among tests are not so large. In the literature, Stone's test is known to have less power compared with other tests via simulation studies; however, the result that Stone's MLR test has the minimum p-value is interesting.

8.5.1.2 Infant Deaths Around MSW Incinerator B

From Table 8.3 we can observe that the trend of O/E ratios for infant deaths around the MSW incinerator B has a "peak" at the 1–2 km zone, and therefore the test statistics designed only for "decline in risk with distance" are expected to be less powerful than those that take "peak-decline in risk with distance" into account. To these data, let us apply six test statistics, including Kulldorff's spatial scan statistic with $N_{rep} = 9999$, using the R codes explained in the previous section. Although we omit the details of the R codes, the results are as follows:

1. Stone's MLR test: $T_S = 1.901, p = 0.1456$.

Table 8.3 Observed and expected numbers of infant deaths for each of ten zones, $(j, j+1], j = 0, 1, ..., 9$ km from the municipal solid waste incinerator B in Japan. Also shown are the O/E ratio, Stone's MLE, and estimated p-values based on Monte Carlo testing with 9999 replications for three tests.

	Zones										
	1	2	3	4	5	6	7	8	9	10	Total
Observed n_i	1	3	1	1	1	2	2	2	4	3	20
Expected e_i	0.998	0.724	1.611	1.623	1.270	1.116	1.820	1.377	3.709	5.752	20
O/E ratio	1.002	4.144	0.621	0.616	0.787	1.792	1.099	1.452	1.078	0.522	
Stone's MLE	2.323	2.323	1.038	1.038	1.038	1.038	1.038	1.038	1.038	0.522	

Stone's MLR test: $p = 0.1456$.
Bithell's LRS test with $g_i = 1/d_i$: $p = 0.1545$.
Waller and Lawson's score test with $g_i = 1/d_i$: $p = 0.2018$.
Tango's score test for decline trend: $p = 0.2047$ ($\lambda^* = 4$).
Tango's score test for peak-decline trend: $p = 0.0304$ ($s^* - 2, \lambda^* = 40$).

2. Bithell's LRS test with $g = 1/d$: $T_B = -33.50, p = 0.1545$. For other exposure functions, $g = 1/d^a$, $(a = 0.2, 0.5, 2, 3)$, p-values are almost the same.
3. Waller and Lawson's score test with $g = 1/d$: $T_{WL} = 0.809, p = 0.2018$. For other exposure functions, $g = 1/d^a$, $(a = 0.2, 0.5, 2, 3)$, as the value of a increases, the p-values also increase from 0.1615 to 0.2846.
4. Tango's score test for decline trend: $T_{\text{decline}} = 1.253, p = 0.2047$ ($\lambda^* = 4$).
5. Tango's score test for peak-decline trend: $T_{\text{peak-decline}} = 2.759, p = 0.0304$ ($s^* = 2, \lambda^* = 40$).
6. Kulldorff's spatial scan statistic (for hot-spot trend): MLC $= 0 - 2$ km zone with $p = 0.1983$.

As expected, Tango's score test for peak-decline trend only detected significant clustering around the MSW incinerator B with estimated peak in the $1 - 2$ km zone.

8.5.2 Leukemia Cases Near Inactive Hazardous Waste Sites

These data have already been described and analyzed using general tests for spatial clustering in subsection 5.5.2. The data are 592 incident leukemia cases from 1978 to 1982 for each of 790 census tracts among 1,057,673 people at risk in an eight-county region of upstate New York. There were 11 inactive hazardous waste sites containing TCE (trichloroethylene) in this area. Exposure to TCE was a motivating concern in the epidemiological study. Locations of inactive hazardous waste sites S1,..., S11 were shown in Figure 5.14. Table 8.4 gives the results of the six focused tests applied to five inactive hazardous waste sites using R codes described previously. The results suggest statistically significant clustering around these sites. Regarding comparison of tests, Bithell's LRS test performs very well except for the

Table 8.4 Results of the six focused tests applied to five inactive hazardous waste sites in New York. All the p-values are based on Monte Carlo testing with 9999 replications.

	Site				
	S1	S2	S3	S5	S8
	Monarch	IBM	Singer	GE	Victory
	Chemicals	Endicott		Auburn	Plaza
Bithell's LRS test (1/d)	0.0004	0.0004	0.0002	0.5205	0.0005
Bithell's LRS test (1/rank)	0.0004	0.0004	0.0002	0.6958	0.0004
Waller and Lawson's score (1/d)	0.0001	0.0010	0.0033	0.0257	0.0131
Waller and Lawson's score ($1/d^2$)	0.0002	0.0139	0.0875	0.0822	0.1082
Tango's score (decline)	0.0004	0.0009	0.0013	0.0128	0.0444
Tango's score (peak-decline)	0.0003	0.0004	0.0012	0.0159	0.0272
	($s^* = 2$)	($s^* = 2$)	($s^* = 2$)	($s^* = 0$)	($s^* = 6$)

site GE Auburn. Tango's score tests with decline trend and peak-decline trend also perform very well.

8.5.3 Larynx and Lung Cancer Near a Disused Incinerator

Diggle (1990), Diggle and Rowlingson (1994), and Diggle, Morris, and Morton-Jones (1999) illustrate their method with data consisting of the residential location of cases of lung and larynx cancers near a now disused industrial incinerator in the Chorley-Ribble area of Lancashire, England. The data set used here is taken from the library Splancs implemented in the statistical software package R, where there are 917 controls and 57 cases in this data set shown in Figure 8.1; these numbers differ from 978 and 58 in Diggle (1990) and Diggle and Rowlingson (1994). The data set also includes the approximate location of an old incinerator, as well as the study area boundary. To this data set also, let us take two approaches. One is to apply tests for count data by dividing the study area into ten plus one zones delimited by ten circles of radii 1, 2,..., 10 km. The eleventh zone denote the outer region of the circle with radius 10 km. The other approach is the application of Diggle, Morris, and Morton-Jones' test using raw case-control individual locations.

8.5.3.1 Analysis Based on 11 Zones

Results of five focused tests are shown in Table 8.5. All the tests except for Bithell's LRS test detect significant clustering around the incinerator at significance level 0.05. Especially, Tango's score test performs very well.

Table 8.5 Observed and expected numbers of infant deaths for each of 11 zones, $(j, j + 1], j = 0, 1, ..., 9$ and $(10, -]$ km from a now disused industrial incinerator in the Chorley-Ribble area of Lancashire, England (Diggle, 1990). Also shown are the O/E ratio, Stone's MLE, and estimated p-values based on Monte Carlo testing with 9999 replications for five tests.

	Zones											
	1	2	3	4	5	6	7	8	9	10	11	Total
Observed cases n_i	4	1	1	2	6	6	2	4	5	2	24	57
Cases+ controls	9	24	12	65	115	114	40	73	120	33	369	917
Expected e_i	0.527	1.405	0.702	3.804	6.730	6.671	2.341	4.272	7.022	1.931	21.594	
O/E ratio	7.595	0.712	1.424	0.526	0.892	0.899	0.854	0.936	0.712	1.036	1.111	
Stone's MLE	7.594	0.949	0.949	0.938	0.938	0.938	0.938	0.938	0.938	0.938	0.938	

Stone's MLR test: $p = 0.0118$.
Bithell's LRS test with $g_i = 1/d_i$: $p = 0.0903$.
Waller and Lawson's score test with $g_i = 1/d_i$: $p = 0.0051$.
Tango's score test for decline trend: $p = 0.0011$ $(\lambda^* = 2)$.
Tango's score test for peak-decline trend: $p = 0.0013$ $(s^* = 0, \lambda^* = 2)$.

8.5.3.2 Analysis Based on Individual Locations

Let us apply Diggle, Morris, and Morton-Jones' test for case-control point data to this data set. To do this, we write a program in Fortran instead of R in order to reduce the computing time. Figure 8.2 shows the isotonic regression estimate of $\theta_{(i)} = \Pr\{Y_{(i)} = 1\}$, the probability that an individual (i) is a case, as a function of distance from the incinerator. The test of significance of the null hypothesis of constant risk against the alternative hypothesis of decline in risk with distance from the incinerator gives an observed test statistic $T_D = 20.02$ with p-value of 0.001 based on the Monte Carlo hypothesis test with $N_{rep} = 999$.

8.6 Power Comparison

In this section, we shall compare powers of six different tests, Stone's MLR test, Bithell's LRS test with inverse of distance, Bithell's LRS test with reciprocal of distance rank, Waller and Lawson's score test with inverse of distance, Tango's score test for decline trend, and Tango's score test with peak-decline trend, using hypothetical regional count data via Monte Carlo simulation. As an entire study area, we shall consider $m = 113$ regions comprising the wards, cities, and villages in the Tokyo metropolis and the Kanagawa prefecture in Japan as an entire study population. The variability of regional populations for the 113 regions is 25th percentile $= 56,704$, median$= 142,320$ and 75th percentile $= 200,936$. In Figure 8.3, 113 circles with various sizes are plotted. The center of a circle is the location of the population centroid of the corresponding region, and the radius is proportional to the square root of the population size, so that the area of each circle is proportional to the pop-

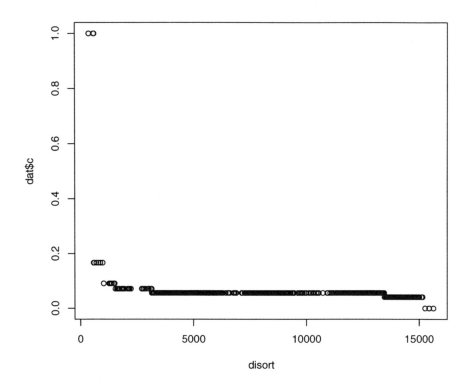

Fig. 8.2 The isotonic regression estimate of the probability that an individual is a case as a function of distance from the incinerator.

ulation size. The distance d_{ij} between any two regions was calculated in kilometers using the approximate formula applicable to the Tokyo metropolitan area

$$d_{ij} = \sqrt{90.15^2(x_i - x_j)^2 + 110.9^2(y_i - y_j)^2} \quad \text{(in km)}$$

where x_i and y_i indicate the longitude and latitude of the geographical population centroid of the ith region and the constants 90.15 and 110.9 serve to transform longitude and latitude to kilometers (for Japan). The maximum and minimum distances between regions are 93.82 km and 1.58 km, respectively.

Clustering model

We shall consider here the following three models of focused clusters: (a) a decline model, (b) a hot-spot model, and (c) a hot-spot model with a shifted peak.

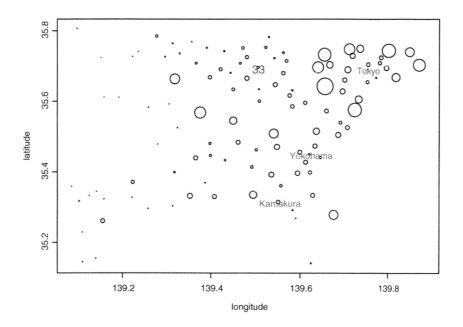

Fig. 8.3 The 113 regions comprising wards, cities, and villages in the areas of the Tokyo metropolis and Kanagawa prefecture in Japan. The center of a circle is the location of the population centroid of the corresponding region, and the area of the circle is set proportional to the population size. The point source to be used in the simulation is indicated by region number "33".

1. *Decline models*

   In this model, one point source is located in region 33, which is illustrated in Figure 8.3. The location of the point source is approximated by the centroid of the region including it, and the true relative risks are assumed to be

$$\theta_i = 1 + (RR - 1)\exp(-d_i/5), \quad RR = 2,3,4 \tag{8.27}$$

   Figure 8.4 illustrates that a clinal cluster with $RR = 3$ occurred around region 33, in which the area of each circle is set proportional to the relative risk assumed.

2. *Hot-spot models*

   The location of the point source is the same as that for decline models. The true relative risks are set as

$$\theta_i = \begin{cases} RR, \text{ if } d_i \leq 5 \text{ km}, \quad RR = 2,3,4 \\ \\ 1.0, \text{ otherwise} \end{cases} \tag{8.28}$$

3. *Hot-spot models with a shifted peak*

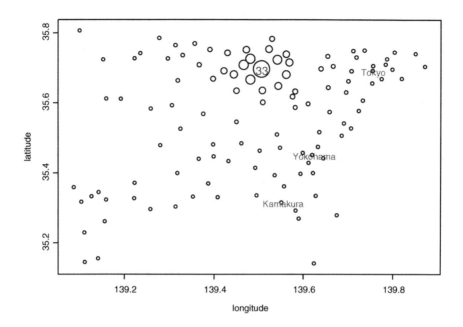

Fig. 8.4 The assumed cluster model with relative risk defined in equation (8.27) around region 33. The area of the circle is set proportional to the relative risk assumed.

The location of the point source is the same as that for decline models. However, the peak of risk is not on the point source but on an area at some distance from the point source. Then, the true relative risks are set as

$$
\theta_i = \begin{cases} RR, \text{ if } 3 \leq d_i \leq 5 \text{ km}, \quad RR = 2,3,4 \\ \\ 1.0, \text{ otherwise} \end{cases} \tag{8.29}
$$

Monte Carlo simulation

The same null hypothesis is used throughout, where the relative risk is set to one for each region and case locations are independent of each other. Although the N_i's are independent Poisson random variables, by conditioning on the total number of cases $N_+ = n$, the disease locations are the values of a random sample of size n from a multinomial distribution with parameter (8.6). We generated 10,000 random data sets with n cases, and these are used to estimate the upper 5% point and 1% point for significance. Under each alternative hypothesis, we generated 1000 random data sets with n cases. In this simulation, we consider the case $n = 200$.

Table 8.6 Estimated power of tests of nominal α levels of 0.05 and 0.01 from 1000 trials of simulation in the case of one point source. Bold numbers indicate the maximum power.

Cluster type	α level	Test statistics	RR 2	3	4
Decline	0.05	Stone's MLR	30.4	68.8	90.9
		Bithell's LRS $(1/d)$	39.0	78.6	95.1
		Bithell's LRS (1/rank)	**39.6**	**79.7**	**95.6**
		Waller and Lawson's score $(1/d)$	29.2	56.6	77.9
		Tango's score (decline)	38.4	77.4	94.6
		Tango's score (peak-decline)	37.9	76.1	94.1
	0.01	Stone's MLR	12.6	45.9	78.4
		Bithell's LRS $(1/d)$	16.9	54.3	84.3
		Bithell's LRS (1/rank)	**17.4**	**55.5**	**85.7**
		Waller and Lawson's score $(1/d)$	11.3	32.4	55.8
		Tango's score (decline)	15.5	52.3	82.9
		Tango's score (peak-decline)	14.9	49.0	80.5
Hot spot $(d \leq 5\ \text{km})$	0.05	Stone's MLR	41.9	86.8	98.4
		Bithell's LRS $(1/d)$	40.5	80.5	95.9
		Bithell's LRS (1/rank)	45.6	85.6	97.6
		Waller and Lawson's score $(1/d)$	34.8	68.7	88.4
		Tango's score (decline)	52.3	91.4	99.1
		Tango's score (peak-decline)	**55.0**	**93.7**	**99.6**
	0.01	Stone's MLR	21.3	71.4	95.2
		Bithell's LRS $(1/d)$	18.8	58.3	87.3
		Bithell's LRS (1/rank)	21.9	66.2	91.9
		Waller and Lawson's score $(1/d)$	14.8	44.1	72.3
		Tango's score (decline)	28.2	77.8	96.8
		Tango's score (peak-decline)	**31.2**	**80.3**	**98.6**
Hot spot $(3 \leq d \leq 5\ \text{km})$	0.05	Stone's MLR	22.4	55.1	85.0
		Bithell's LRS $(1/d)$	20.3	47.2	73.3
		Bithell's LRS (1/rank)	24.3	56.0	82.9
		Waller and Lawson's score $(1/d)$	8.3	13.7	19.1
		Tango's score (decline)	24.2	57.3	84.8
		Tango's score (peak-decline)	**27.2**	**63.5**	**90.6**
	0.01	Stone's MLR	7.6	34.5	68.1
		Bithell's LRS $(1/d)$	6.3	21.4	46.2
		Bithell's LRS (1/rank)	8.3	27.4	57.8
		Waller and Lawson's score $(1/d)$	1.7	2.8	5.6
		Tango's score (decline)	7.7	31.2	63.1
		Tango's score (peak-decline)	**9.7**	**39.7**	**72.0**

(Note): For Tango's score test for peak-decline trend, we set $s \in \{0, 2, 4, 6, 8\}$ km.

The resultant powers for tests of nominal α levels of 0.05 and 0.01, sample size $n = 200$, and $RR = 2, 3, 4$ are shown in Table 8.6 for each of three cluster models in which we can observe several interesting characteristics of tests.

- Surprisingly, Waller and Lawson's score test with $g_i = 1/d_i$ has the lowest power against all three alternatives considered. This observation is clearly due to the fact that this test is quite sensitive to the selection of the exposure function.
- On the other hand, as the two Tango score tests search for the optimal exposure function, they have good power against all three alternatives considered. Especially, Tango's score test with peak-decline trend (including decline trend) has the largest power against two hot-spot alternatives.
- It is interesting to see that Bithell's LRS test with $g_i = 1/\text{rank}$ has the largest power and Bithell's LRS test with $g_i = 1/d$ has the second largest against decline alternatives.
- Although Stone's MLR test appears to have lower power against decline alternatives, it has good power against two hot-spot alternatives.

Recommendation

Based on the results of illustrative examples and power comparisons performed here and in the literature, we can recommend the following tests:

1. *Regional count data*

   - If we would like to test the null hypothesis against the alternative hypothesis of decline in risk with distance from the point source, we can recommend (a) Bithell's LRS test with $g_i = 1/\text{rank}$ or $1/d$, (b) Tango's score test for decline trend, and (c) Stone's LRT test to estimate its pattern nonparametrically.
   - If we do not have any sufficient information on the pattern of exposure around the point source and we cannot predict any pattern, then Tango's score test for peak-decline trend is the only recommendable test. In this situation, we cannot recommend Stone's MLR test because we cannot assume nonincreasing restriction of (8.9).

2. *Case-control data*

   When we have case-control data around the point source, we would like to recommend the following two approaches as illustrated with data from larynx and lung cancer incidences near a disused incinerator:

   - Apply a test (recommended above) for count data by dividing the study area into several zones; for example, 11 zones delimited by ten circles of radii of 1, 2,..., 10 km. The eleventh zone denotes the outer region of the circle with radius 10 km.
   - Apply Diggle, Morris, and Morton-Jones' test using raw case-control individual locations.

However, the former method will be recommended in terms of ease of interpretation of test results, especially for non-statistical researchers.

Chapter 9
Space-Time Scan Statistics

Tests for *space-time interaction* or *space-time clustering*, described in Chapter 7, are designed for evaluating whether cases tend to come in groups or are located close to each other no matter when and where they occur. *Space-time scan statistics*, on the other hand, are designed for both detecting localized clusters in three dimensional space and evaluating their significance, which are extensions of purely spatial scan statistics. Recently, Kulldorff's (2001) cylindrical space-time scan statistic has been implemented in many syndromic surveillance systems as a major analytical tool for outbreak detection.

Example 1

Figure 9.1 shows the outbreaks of rash and respiratory syndrome in eastern Massachusetts during August 1–30, 2005, detected by the cylindrical scan statistic and the prismatic scan statistic applied to daily syndromic surveillance data (Takahashi *et al.*, 2008).

9.1 Data

To apply the space-time scan statistics, we need to collect data on the location of each case for a defined geographic area during a specified study period. Throughout this chapter, it is assumed that:

1. The total observed number of cases is n.
2. The study area is divided into m_S geographic regions (e.g., census tracts, counties, or states), and the study period is divided into m_T intervals, where:

   a. The observed number of cases of the disease under study in region i at time t is denoted by n_{it} with $n = n_{11} + \cdots + n_{m_S m_T}$.
   b. The conditional null expected number of cases of the disease under study in region i at time t is denoted by e_{it}.

T. Tango, *Statistical Methods for Disease Clustering*,
Statistics for Biology and Health, DOI 10.1007/978-1-4419-1572-6_9,
© Springer Science+Business Media, LLC 2010

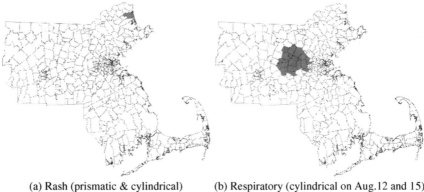

(a) Rash (prismatic & cylindrical)   (b) Respiratory (cylindrical on Aug.12 and 15)

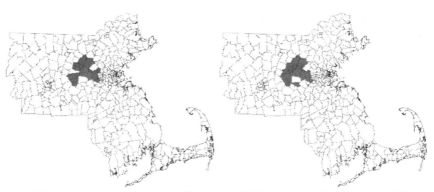

(c) Respiratory (prismatic on Aug.12)   (d) Respiratory (prismatic on Aug.15)

Fig. 9.1 Detected outbreaks of rash and respiratory syndrome in eastern Massachusetts during August 1–30, 2005, by the cylindrical scan statistic ((a) and (b)) and the prismatic scan statistic ((a), (c), and (d)) (Takahashi *et al.*, 2008).

c. To calculate the e_{it} using equation (9.4), we need the observed number of cases n_{itk} and the population size ξ_{itk} in the kth category of the set of confounders of the region i at time t.

d. The centroid of region i is denoted by (x_i, y_i).

e. The distance between the ith and jth regions is defined as d_{ij}
$= \sqrt{(x_i - x_j)^2 + (y_i - y_j)^2}$.

9.2 Null Hypothesis vs. Alternative Hypothesis

We shall consider here only the Poisson model. The null hypothesis of *no clustering in space-time* and the alternative hypothesis can be simply stated as follows:

H_0 : the locations of onset (or diagnosis or death) of the disease under study
are randomly distributed across the study area and study period

H_1 : the locations of onset of the disease under study are clustered within
some space-time (three-dimensional) domain

Statistically speaking, we can restate these hypotheses as follows. Consider the situation where an entire study area is divided into m_S regions and the study period is divided into m_T intervals. The number of cases in region i at time t is denoted by the Poisson random number N_{it} with observed number n_{it}

$$H_0 : \quad N_{it} \sim \text{Independent Poisson}(e'_{it}), \quad (e'_{it} \text{ is usually unknown}) \qquad (9.1)$$

where $i = 1, ..., m_S$, $t = 1, ..., m_T$, and the time interval m_T includes the current time. Then, using the same logic as in Section 5.2, conditioning on the observed total number of cases, $n = \sum_{it} n_{it}$, the null hypothesis of no clustering can be

$$H_0 : \quad E(N_{it}) = e_{it}, \quad (N_{11}, ..., N_{m_S m_T}) \sim \text{Multinomial}(n, \boldsymbol{p}) \qquad (9.2)$$

where

$$\boldsymbol{p} = (p_{11}, p_{12}, ..., p_{m_S m_T})^t, \quad p_{it} = e_{it}/n \qquad (9.3)$$

where e_{it} denotes the *conditional* null expected number of cases in region i at time t adjusted for the confounding factors such as sex and age and is given by

$$e_{it} = \sum_{k=1}^{K} \xi_{itk} \left(\frac{\sum_{j=1}^{m_S} \sum_{t=1}^{m_T} n_{jtk}}{\sum_{j=1}^{m_S} \sum_{t=1}^{m_T} \xi_{jtk}} \right), \quad (i = 1, ..., m_S; t = 1, ..., m_T) \qquad (9.4)$$

where n_{jtk} and ξ_{jtk} denote the observed number of cases and the population size in the kth category of the set of potential confounders of the jth region at time t, respectively. Then we have

$$\sum_{i=1}^{m_S} \sum_{t=1}^{m_T} \sum_{k=1}^{K} n_{itk} = \sum_{i=1}^{m_S} \sum_{t=1}^{m_T} e_{it} = n \qquad (9.5)$$

On the other hand, when we obtain the covariate adjusted expected number of cases e_{it}^R using regression models such as a generalized linear mixed model (for example, see Kleinman, Lazarus and Platt, 2004), the conditional expectation is calculated as

$$e_{it} = \frac{ne_{it}^R}{\sum_{i=1}^{m_S} \sum_{t=1}^{m_T} e_{it}^R} \tag{9.6}$$

so that $\sum_{i=1}^{m_S} \sum_{t=1}^{m_T} e_{it} = n$. In general, we can write

$$E(N_{it}) = \theta_{it} e_{it}, \quad (N_{11}, ..., N_{m_S m_T}) \sim \text{Multinomial} \tag{9.7}$$

where θ_{it} denotes the relative risk due to the region i and the time t. Then, in terms of the relative risks, the null hypothesis can be stated as

$$H_0: \ \theta_{11} = \cdots = \theta_{1 m_T} = \theta_{21} = \cdots = \theta_{2 m_T} = \cdots = \theta_{m_S m_T} = 1 \tag{9.8}$$

Let $W = Z \times I$ denotes some connected space-time domain, Z is a spatial window or base scanning by scan statistics, I is a temporal window, and let us assume a *hot-spot model* such that

$$\theta_{it} = \begin{cases} \theta(W), & \text{if } (i,t) \in W = Z \times I \\ \\ \theta(W^c), & \text{otherwise} \end{cases} \tag{9.9}$$

where W^c denotes all the domains except for W. That is, $\theta(W)$ and $\theta(W^c)$ are assumed to be the common relative risk within the domain W and outside the domain W, respectively. Then, the *ordinary* space-time scan statistics test the following null hypothesis H_0 against the alternative hypothesis H_1 for all possible sets of domains W:

$$H_0: \ \theta(W) = \theta(W^c) \tag{9.10}$$
$$H_1: \ \theta(W) > \theta(W^c) \tag{9.11}$$

The domain W for which the likelihood ratio is maximized identifies the most likely cluster (MLC) as in the case of purely spatial scan statistics. As in the case of spatial scan statistics, to find the distribution of the test statistic under the null hypothesis, Monte Carlo hypothesis testing is required.

The space-time scan statistics may be used for single retrospective analysis and also for time-periodic prospective surveillance, where the analysis is repeated, for example, every day, week, and so on.

9.3 Historical Overview of Methods

(It should be noted that there are several other proposed methods not mentioned here. Furthermore, readers who are not interested in the history can skip this section.)

9.3.1 Retrospective Analysis

Kulldorff *et al.* (1998) proposed the *cylindrical space-time scan statistic* by extending the basic idea of the circular spatial scan statistic to explore brain cancer incidence in Los Alamos, a remote New Mexican community established in 1943. The cylindrical space-time scan statistic uses a cylindrical domain in three dimensions, where the base of the cylinder represents space and the height represents time. As with the purely spatial scan statistic, the cylindrical space-time scan statistic imposes a circular base Z on each centroid of regions for each possible time interval (defined later). For each centroid, the radius of the circle is varied from zero up to a preset maximum radius, for example, so that the domain never includes more than 50% of the total population at risk. We can also use a preset maximum number of regions K to be included in the cluster as an upper bound on the radius. If the base contains the centroid of a region, then that whole region is included in the base. In total, a very large number of different but overlapping circular bases are created, each with a different set of neighboring regions and each being a possible candidate area containing a disease outbreak. Let Z_{ik}, $k = 1, \ldots, K$, denote the base composed of the region i and the $(k-1)$ nearest neighbors to i. Then, all the cylindrical domains to be scanned by the cylindrical scan statistic are the cylinders with base in the set

$$\mathscr{Z}_1 = \{Z_{ik} \mid i = 1, \ldots, m_S, \ k = 1, \ldots, K\}$$

and height in the set of discrete time intervals

$$\mathscr{Y}_1 = \{[u, \ u+v] \mid u = 1, \ldots, m_T, \ v = 0, \ldots, m_T - u\}$$

Define L_0 as the likelihood under the null hypothesis and $L(W)$ as that under the alternative hypothesis that there is a cluster in the space-time domain $W \, (\in \mathscr{W}_1)$, where $\mathscr{W}_1 = \mathscr{Z}_1 \times \mathscr{Y}_1$. Then, conditioning on the observed total number of cases, n, the definition of the space-time scan statistic λ is the *conditional* maximum likelihood ratio over all possible domains W

$$\lambda = \sup_{W \in \mathscr{W}_1} \left\{ \frac{L(W)}{L_0} \right\}$$

$$= \sup_{W \in \mathscr{W}_1} \left(\frac{n(W)}{e(W)} \right)^{n(W)} \left(\frac{n - n(W)}{n - e(W)} \right)^{n - n(W)} I\left(\frac{n(W)}{e(W)} > \frac{n - n(W)}{n - e(W)} \right)$$

where $I()$ is the indicator function and $n()$ and $e()$ denote the observed number of cases and the *conditional* null expected number of cases within the specified domain, respectively,

$$n(W) = \sum_{(i,t) \in W} n_{it}$$

$$e(W) = \sum_{(i,t) \in W} e_{it}$$

The domain for which the *conditional* likelihood ratio is maximized identifies the most likely cluster (MLC). To find the distribution of the space-time scan statistic λ under the null hypothesis, Monte Carlo hypothesis testing is required. There may also be secondary clusters that do not overlap with the MLC that may be of great interest. The *p*-value of the secondary clusters is obtained by comparing the likelihood of secondary clusters with that of the MLC in Monte Carlo simulated data.

The cylindrical space-time scan statistic is implemented in SaTScan. Applications of the cylindrical space-time scan statistic include childhood malignant brain tumors in Sweden (Hjalmars *et al.*, 1999), soft-tissue sarcomas, non-Hodgkin's lymphomas and Hodgkin's disease around a solid waste incinerator in France (Viel *et al.*, 2000), anthrax strains in Kruger National Park in South Africa (Smith *et al.*, 2000), and breast cancer in western Massachusetts (Sheehan and De Chello, 2005).

9.3.2 Syndromic Surveillance

The anthrax terrorist attacks in 2001, the severe acute respiratory syndrome (SARS) outbreak in 2002, and a concern about pandemic influenza have motivated many public health departments to develop early disease outbreak detection systems. Early detection of disease outbreaks enables public health officials to implement disease control and prevention measures at the earliest possible time (for example, see Sonesson and Bock, 2003; Lawson and Kleinman, 2005). For an infectious disease, improvement in detection time by even one day might enable public health officials to control the disease before it becomes widespread. In many cities such as New York City (Heffernan *et al.*, 2004), Washington, D.C. (Lombardo *et al.*, 2003), Boston (Lazarus *et al.*, 2002; Platt *et al.*, 2003), Denver, and Minneapolis, real-time, geographic, early outbreak detection systems have been implemented.

Kulldorff (2001) proposed the prospective use of the cylindrical space-time scan statistic as part of a time-periodic geographical disease surveillance system to detect the locations of emerging clusters and evaluate their significance, where the set of heights includes only m_T intervals of discrete time points including current time t_p

$$\mathcal{U}_2 = \{I_1, ..., I_{m_T}\}$$

where

$$I_u = [t_p - u + 1, \ t_p] \quad (u = 1, \cdots, m_T)$$

where m_T is a prespecified *maximum temporal length* of the cluster. Then, domains to be scanned are restricted to the set

$$\mathscr{W}_2 = \mathscr{Z}_1 \times \mathscr{Y}_2$$

instead of $\mathscr{W}_1$ used in the retrospective analysis.

Takahashi *et al.* (2008), on the other hand, proposed a *prismatic space-time scan statistic* by extending Tango and Takahashi's (2005) flexible spatial scan statistic, which imposes a three-dimensional prismatic domain with an arbitrarily shaped base Z. For any given region i, we create the set of arbitrarily shaped bases consisting of k connected regions ($1 \leq k \leq K$) including i. To avoid detecting a cluster of unlikely peculiar shape, the connected regions are restricted as the subset of the K nearest neighbors to the region i, where $K = 1$ implies the region i itself. Let $Z_{ik(j)}$, $j = 1, \ldots, j_{ik}$, denotes the jth spatial window that is a set of k regions connected starting from the region i, where j_{ik} is the number of j's satisfying $Z_{ik(j)} \subseteq Z_{iK}$ for $k = 1, \ldots, K$. In other words, for any given region i, the cylindrical scan statistic considers K concentric circles for the base, whereas the flexible scan statistic consider K concentric circles plus all the sets of connected regions, including the single region i, whose centroids are located within the Kth-largest concentric circle. Then, all the domains to be scanned are the *prisms* whose base is included in the set

$$\mathscr{Z}_2 = \{ Z_{ik(j)} \mid i = 1, \ldots, m_S, \ k = 1, \ldots, K, \ j = 1, \ldots, j_{ik} \}$$

with the heights in the set $\mathscr{Y}_1$ if the study is retrospective and in the set $\mathscr{Y}_2$ if the study is prospective. These two kinds of space-time scan statistics considered the *right* cylinder or *right* prism of the cluster model, which cannot model growth, shrinkage, or movement of the disease cluster over time. Iyengar (2005) suggests using the *square pyramid shape*, which can model growth (or shrinkage) and movement of the disease cluster.

For the above-mentioned space-time scan statistics, we have assumed that data on the population at risk ξ_{itk} are available. However, there could be a situation where such population data are not available. Kulldorff *et al.* (2005) proposed a *cylindrical space-time permutation scan statistic* for the early detection of disease outbreaks that uses only case numbers, with no need for population-at-risk data. It makes minimal assumptions about the time, geographical location, or size of the outbreak, and it adjusts for natural purely spatial and purely temporal variations. Suppose we have daily case counts for zip-code areas, where n_{it} is the observed number of cases in zip-code area i during day t. However, calculation of the expected number of cases e_{it} is totally different. Since we do not have population-at-risk data, the expected number of cases must be calculated using only the cases assuming the steady state; i.e., the population increase or decrease is the same across the study region. For each zip code and day, we calculate the expected number of cases e_{it} conditioning on the observed marginals:

$$e_{it} = \frac{\left(\sum_{i=1}^{m_S} n_{it} \right) \left(\sum_{t=1}^{m_T} n_{it} \right)}{n}$$

In other words, this number would have been expected if the spatial and temporal locations of all cases were independent of each other so that there was no space-time interaction. Conditioned on the marginals, and when there is no space-time interaction, $n(W)$ for a particular cylinder W is distributed according to the hypergeometric distribution

$$\Pr\{N(W) = n(W)\} = \binom{\sum_{i \in W} n_{it}}{n(W)} \binom{n - \sum_{i \in W} n_{it}}{\sum_{t \in W} n_{it} - n(W)} \bigg/ \binom{n}{\sum_{t \in W} n_{it}}$$

When both $\sum_{i \in W} n_{it}$ and $\sum_{t \in W} n_{it}$ are small compared with n, $N(W)$ is approximately Poisson distributed with mean $e(W) = \sum_{(i,t) \in W} e_{it}$. Based on this approximation, Kulldorff *et al.* (2005) used the Poisson generalized likelihood ratio (GLR) as a measure of the evidence that the cylindrical domain W contains an outbreak:

$$\left(\frac{n(W)}{e(W)} \right)^{n(W)} \left(\frac{n - n(W)}{n - e(W)} \right)^{n - n(W)}$$

Among the many domains evaluated, the one with the maximum GLR constitutes the space-time cluster of cases that is least likely to be a chance occurrence and hence is the primary candidate for a true outbreak. To find the distribution of the maximum GLR under the null hypothesis, Monte Carlo hypothesis testing is also required. However, since we do not have population-at-risk data, this cannot be done in any of the usual ways for spatial scan statistics. Instead, it is done by creating a large number of random permutations of the spatial and temporal attributes of each case in the data set. That is, we shuffle the dates and times and assign them to the original set of case locations, ensuring that both the spatial and temporal marginals are unchanged. This randomization is not so easy and requires a special computational technique. After that, the most likely cluster is calculated for each simulated data set in exactly the same way as for the real data. Kulldorff *et al.* (2005) evaluated the space-time permutation scan statistic using daily analyses of hospital emergency department visits in New York City. Four of the five strongest signals were likely local precursors to citywide outbreaks due to rotavirus, norovirus, and influenza. The number of false signals was at most modest.

In syndromic surveillance, the null occurrence rate or recurrence interval (RI) is often used as an alternative to the *p*-value (Kleinman, Lazarus, and Platt, 2004). The measure reflects how often a cluster will be observed by chance, assuming that analyses are repeated on a regular basis with a periodicity equal to the period of the study. For daily surveillance such as this analysis, the *p*-value of 0.001 corresponds to the RI of 1000 days (i.e., 2.7 years), and an alpha level of 0.0027 corresponds to one expected false alarm every year.

Note

It should be noted that all the *prospective* space-time scan statistics described so far compare the observed number of cases with the *conditional* expected number of cases e_{it} such as those defined in (9.4) or (9.6). Therefore, the most likely cluster detected by space-time scan statistics introduced so far will not always be *emerging outbreak*. To detect *emerging outbreak* more correctly, the observed number of cases should be compared with the number of cases *unconditionally* expected from data in the baseline periods for outbreak detection. Kleinman *et al.* (2005) proposed a space-time scan statistic based on the expected number of cases adjusted for naturally occurring temporal trends or geographical patterns in illness using the model discussed in Kleinman, Lazarus, and Platt (2004). However, their space-time scan statistic still uses the *conditional* expected number of cases (9.6). Similar arguments can be applied to the cylindrical space-time permutation scan statistic. For details and other related problems associated with prospective space-time scan statistics, see Section 9.7.

9.4 Selected Methods

Although we describe here two space-time scan statistics derived under the Poisson model (Kulldorff's and Takahashi *et al's*), we have to resort to statistical software to make practical use of these computationally intensive methods.

9.4.1 Kulldorff's Cylindrical Space-Time Scan Statistic

Goal: To detect the most likely *cylindrical* hot-spot cluster and secondary clusters, if any, within the study area and during the study period and evaluate its (their) statistical significance. The finding that the most likely cluster is significant would suggest evidence for the occurrence of a localized cylindrical cluster or emerging outbreak.

Test statistic (under Poisson model)

$$\lambda = \sup_{W \in \mathscr{W}} \left(\frac{n(W)}{e(W)} \right)^{n(W)} \left(\frac{n - n(W)}{n - e(W)} \right)^{n - n(W)} I\left(\frac{n(W)}{e(W)} > \frac{n - n(W)}{n - e(W)} \right) \quad (9.12)$$

where W denotes the cylindrical domain and

$$n(W) = \sum_{(i,t) \in W} n_{it}, \quad e(W) = \sum_{(i,t) \in W} e_{it} \quad (9.13)$$

The cylindrical domain $\boldsymbol{W}$ to be scanned by the space-time scan statistic is included in the set

$$\mathscr{W} = \begin{cases} \mathscr{W}_1 = \mathscr{Z}_1 \times \mathscr{Y}_1, \text{ for retropective use} \\ \\ \mathscr{W}_2 = \mathscr{Z}_1 \times \mathscr{Y}_2, \text{ for prospective surveillance} \end{cases} \quad (9.14)$$

where

$$\mathscr{Z}_1 = \{\mathbf{Z}_{ik} \mid i = 1, ..., m_S, \ k = 1, ..., K_i\} \tag{9.15}$$

$$\mathscr{Y}_1 = \{[u, u+v] \mid u = 1, ..., m_T, \ v = 0, ..., m_T - u\} \tag{9.16}$$

$$\mathscr{Y}_2 = \{I_0, I_1, ..., I_{m_T - 1}\} \tag{9.17}$$

$$I_u = [t_p - u + 1, t_p] \quad (u = 1, ..., m_T) \tag{9.18}$$

where $\mathbf{Z}_{ik}$, $k = 1, ..., K_i$, denotes the base of the cylinder composed by the $(k-1)$ nearest neighbors to region i, the interval $[u, u+v]$ represents the height of the cylinder, and m_T is a prespecified *maximum temporal length* of the cluster. The value of K_i depends on the starting region i so that the radius of the circle varies from zero upward until 50% of the total population is covered. The cylindrical domain $\mathbf{W}^*$ with (Z^*, u^*, v^*) or (Z^*, u^*) that attains the maximum likelihood ratio is defined as the *most likely cluster* (MLC). If the most likely cluster is significant, then we can search for significant *secondary clusters* that do not overlap with the most likely cluster, if any, and order them according to their likelihood ratio test statistic.

Null distribution

Monte Carlo hypothesis testing is required to obtain the null distribution of λ and the Monte Carlo simulated p-value (2.17). The p-value of a secondary cluster is obtained by comparing its likelihood with the null distribution of λ.

Software

SaTScan: http://www.satscan.org/

9.4.2 Takahashi et al.'s Prismatic Space-Time Scan Statistic

Goal: To detect the most likely *prismatic* hot-spot cluster and secondary clusters, if any, within the study area and during the study period and evaluate its (their) statistical significance. The finding that the most likely cluster is significant would suggest evidence for the occurrence of a localized prismatic cluster or emerging outbreak.

Test statistic (under Poisson model)

$$\lambda = \sup_{W \in \mathscr{W}} \left(\frac{n(\mathbf{W})}{e(\mathbf{W})}\right)^{n(\mathbf{W})} \left(\frac{n - n(\mathbf{W})}{n - e(\mathbf{W})}\right)^{n - n(\mathbf{W})} I\left(\frac{n(\mathbf{W})}{e(\mathbf{W})} > \frac{n - n(\mathbf{W})}{n - e(\mathbf{W})}\right) \tag{9.19}$$

where W is a prismatic domain and

$$n(W) = \sum_{(i,t) \in W} n_{it}, \quad e(W) = \sum_{(i,t) \in W} e_{it} \tag{9.20}$$

The prismatic domain $\boldsymbol{W}$ to be scanned by the space-time scan statistic is included in the set

$$\mathcal{W} = \begin{cases} \mathcal{W}_1 = \mathcal{Z}_2 \times \mathcal{Y}_1, \text{ for retrospective use} \\ \\ \mathcal{W}_2 = \mathcal{Z}_2 \times \mathcal{Y}_2, \text{ for prospective surveillance} \end{cases} \tag{9.21}$$

where

$$\mathcal{Z}_2 = \{Z_{ik(j)} \mid i = 1, ..., m_S, \; k = 1, ..., K, \; j = 1, ..., j_{ik}\} \tag{9.22}$$

$$\mathcal{Y}_1 = \{[u, u+v] \mid u = 1, ..., m_T, \; v = 0, ..., m_T - u\} \tag{9.23}$$

$$\mathcal{Y}_2 = \{I_0, I_1, ..., I_{m_T-1}\} \tag{9.24}$$

$$I_u = [t_p - u + 1, t_p] \quad (u = 1, ..., m_T) \tag{9.25}$$

where $\boldsymbol{Z}_{ik(j)}$, $j = 1, \ldots, j_{ik}$, denotes the jth base of the prismatic window that is a set of k regions connected starting from the region i, and j_{ik} is the number of j's satisfying $\boldsymbol{Z}_{ik(j)} \subseteq \boldsymbol{Z}_{ik}$ for $k = 1, \ldots, K_i = K$. Similarly to the flexible spatial scan statistic, the prismatic space-time scan statistic has a limitation of cluster size K that is usually set at 15 or 20. However, $K = 20$ may be large enough for the purpose of an early detection of outbreaks because the outbreak usually starts locally and within a relatively small area. The prismatic domain $\boldsymbol{W}^*$ with (Z^*, u^*, v^*) or (Z^*, u^*) that attains the maximum likelihood ratio is defined as the *most likely cluster* (MLC). If the most likely cluster is significant, then we can search for significant *secondary clusters* that do not overlap with the most likely cluster, if any, and order them according to their likelihood ratio test statistic.

Null distribution

Monte Carlo hypothesis testing is required to obtain the null distribution of λ and the Monte Carlo simulated p-value (2.17). The p-value of a secondary cluster is obtained by comparing its likelihood with the null distribution of λ.

Software

FleXScan: http://www.niph.go.jp/soshiki/gijutsu/download/flexscan/index.html

9.5 Illustration with Real Data

We shall illustrate two space-time scan statistics with daily syndromic surveillance data in Massachusetts, part of the results are shown in Figure 9.1. However, as we cannot show the raw data here we shall only cite some results from Takahashi *et al.* (2008).

Table 9.1 Detected outbreaks of Rash based on daily syndromic surveillance data in eastern Massachusetts during August 1–30, 2005 (Takahashi *et al.*, 2008).

Day	Zip codes	Cluster period	Cases	Expectd	log-likelihood ratio	RI (*p*-value)
Rash:						
– prismatic						
Aug 07	01951	Aug 02–07	7	0.0427	27.949	2.7 years (0.001)
Aug 08	01951	Aug 02–08	7	0.0545	26.259	2.7 years (0.001)
Aug 09	01951	Aug 03–09	6	0.0545	21.562	2.7 years (0.001)
Aug 10	01951	Aug 04–10	5	0.0545	17.315	2.7 years (0.001)
– cylindrical						
Aug 07	01951	Aug 02–07	7	0.0427	27.949	2.7 years (0.001)
Aug 08	01951	Aug 02–08	7	0.0545	26.259	2.7 years (0.001)
Aug 09	01951	Aug 03–09	6	0.0545	21.562	2.7 years (0.001)
Aug 10	01951	Aug 04–10	5	0.0545	17.315	2.7 years (0.001)

9.5.1 Syndromic Surveillance of the Massachusetts Data

Takahashi *et al.* (2008) applied the prospective prismatic space-time scan statistic to daily syndromic surveillance data in eastern Massachusetts mimicking a real-time surveillance system. The data came from an electronic medical record system used by Harvard Vanguard Medical Associates (Lazarus *et al.*, 2001, 2002). They used the rash and respiratory data during August 1–30, 2005. The data are geographically aggregated to zip codes. The number of zip codes used was different for each syndrome; for example, cases of the rash were analyzed in 252 zip codes and respiratory cases in 385. Note that for the prismatic space-time scan statistic, the zip code whose data do not exist was treated like a ravine. For example, assume that zip codes i_1 and i_2, and i_2 and i_3 are adjacent to each other, respectively, but i_1 and i_3 are not adjacent. If the data of i_2 do not exist under the situation, then it is assumed that i_1 and i_3 are not directly connected.

Based on the prior daily data for over a year in MA, the expected number of cases e_{it}^R was calculated as the predicted mean from a generalized linear mixed model (GLMM) as developed by Kleinman *et al.* (2005), adjusted for seasonal effect, day of week, etc. These are the same expectations used in the actual real-time surveillance system (Kleinman, Lazarus, and Platt, 2004). We set $K = 20$ as the maximum length of the geographical window and the maximum temporal length to be $T = 7$ days. The number of replications for the Monte Carlo procedure was set to $N_{rep} = 999$. The results of an analysis during August 1–30 using the prismatic and cylindrical space-time scan statistics are given in Tables 9.1 and 9.2 and Figure 9.1. The tables show results for the days with $p < 0.0054$, which corresponds to an RI of at least 6 months.

When looking at rash outbreaks (Table 9.1), both tests detected the same cluster with the single zip code 01951 on August 7, with the same temporal length (6 days) and the same RI (2.7 years). Note that the clusters detected by both tests from August

Table 9.2 Detected outbreaks of respiratory syndrome based on daily syndromic surveillance data in eastern Massachusetts during August 1–30, 2005 (Takahashi et al., 2008).

Day	Zip codes	Cluster period	Cases	Expected	log-likelihood ratio	RI (p-value)
Respiratory:						
– prismatic						
Aug 12	01720, 01742, 01752, 01754, 01772, 01775, 01776, 01778, 02451, 02462, 02481, 02493	Aug 11–12	42	12.452	17.635	2.7 years (0.001)
Aug 13	01720, 01742, 01749, 01752, 01754, 01772, 01775, 01776, 01778, 02451, 02462, 02481, 02493	Aug 11–13	46	14.950	16.634	333 days (0.003)
Aug 14	01720, 01742, 01749, 01752, 01754, 01772, 01775, 01776, 01778, 02451, 02462, 02481, 02493	Aug 11–14	49	16.957	15.927	250 days (0.004)
Aug 15	01702, 01720, 01742, 01749, 01752, 01754, 01772, 01775, 01776, 01778, 02481, 02493	Aug 10–15	72	29.975	16.726	1.4 years (0.002)
– cylindrical						
Aug 12	01701, 01702, 01718, 01719, 01720, 01742, 01749, 01752, 01754, 01772, 01773, 01775, 01776, 01778, 02451, 02453, 02481, 02493	Aug 11–12	51	20.036	12.688	2.7 years (0.001)
Aug 13	01701, 01702, 01718, 01719, 01720, 01742, 01749, 01752, 01754, 01772, 01773, 01775, 01776, 01778, 02451, 02453, 02481, 02493	Aug 11–13	55	23.768	10.945	91 days (0.011)
Aug 14	01701, 01702, 01718, 01719, 01720, 01742, 01749, 01752, 01754, 01772, 01773, 01775, 01776, 01778, 02451, 02453, 02481, 02493	Aug 11–14	59	26.959	10.221	30 days (0.033)
Aug 15	01701, 01702, 01718, 01719, 01720, 01742, 01749, 01752, 01754, 01772, 01773, 01775, 01776, 01778, 02451, 02453, 02481, 02493	Aug 11–15	82	40.981	11.662	200 days (0.005)

8 to 10 are not signals of an outbreak because the number of cases on August 8 must be 0, and on August 9 and 10 the number of cases of the cluster was decreasing. For respiratory syndrome (Table 9.2), each test detected a different cluster with the same RI of 2.7 years on August 12. The cluster detected by the prismatic scan statistic contained 12 zip codes, while that from the cylindrical scan statistic contained 18 zip codes, with 11 zip codes detected in common. On August 13 and 14, the prismatic scan statistic detected significant clusters with larger RIs, 333 days and 250 days, respectively, while the cylindrical scan statistic detected clusters with short RIs, 91 days and 30 days, respectively. The prismatic scan statistic also detected a cluster on August 15 (RI = 1.4 years) with a temporal length of 6 days, while the cylindrical scan statistic detected a cluster with a temporal length of 5 days (RI = 200 days).

For the six days from August 12 to 17 (results on August 16 and 17 are not shown in Table 9.2 because of shorter RIs), the cylindrical scan statistic kept detecting the same cluster, while the prismatic scan statistic detected a similar but slightly different cluster each day. However, we should acknowledge the similar lack of evidence in Table 9.2 for a continued outbreak on August 13 and 14 because the number of additional cases on those days is very close to the expected number of additional cases. On the other hand, there is some evidence for an excess of cases on August 15 (23 additional cases), although the estimated relative risk is substantially reduced.

9.6 Power Comparison

Takahashi *et al.* (2008) also compare the performance of the prismatic space-time scan statistic with that of the cylindrical scan statistic using benchmark data and a space-time *trivariate* power distribution by extending the purely spatial bivariate power distribution (5.22). The results are summarized as follows: (1) the cylindrical scan statistic performs better for a small and compact cluster and (2) the prismatic scan statistic performs better than the cylindrical one for the large and irregular-shaped cluster. These results are quite similar to the results of comparing Kulldorff's circular spatial scan statistic and Tango and Takahashi's flexible spatial scan statistic.

9.7 Discussion with a New Proposal

As far as I know, the existing *prospective* space-time scan statistics based on the Poisson model assume the basic model (9.7), which is given here again:

$$E(N_{it}) = \theta_{it} e_{it}, \quad (N_{11}, ..., N_{m_S m_T}) \sim \text{Multinomial}$$

However, there are at least the following three problems:

1. **Temporal overdispersion**: In the basic model above, a region-specific time-to-time variation of Poisson mean, so-called overdispersion, cannot be taken into account. As I have already indicated, Kleinman et al. (2005) proposed a space-time scan statistic based on the expected number of cases e_{it}^R adjusted for naturally occurring temporal trends or geographical patterns in illness using the generalized linear mixed model that takes overdispersion into account (Kleinman, Lazarus, and Platt, 2004). However, the region-specific time-to-time variation of the Poisson mean is completely different from the random-effect term introduced in their model.

2. **Calculation of** e_{it}: The *conditional* null expected number of cases defined in (9.4) or (9.6) is used. However, this is not always appropriate for the purpose of detecting emerging outbreak. We have to compare the observed number of cases with the *unconditional* null expected number of cases estimated by baseline data using some kind of generalized linear regression model.

3. **Modeling** θ_{it}: A *hot-spot* cluster was assumed for *an emerging outbreak*. Intuitively, this model would lead to low power or a false alarm because the temporal pattern of emerging outbreaks usually has a *gradual or steep increase* in the number of cases under study. The hot-spot pattern is a special case of temporal patterns of emerging outbreaks.

Tango and Takahashi (2008) recently proposed a new cylindrical/prismatic space-time scan statistic to cope with the problem stated above, which was presented at the 7th Annual International Society for Disease Surveillance Conference. Their model is described below and is illustrated with data from weekly surveillance on the number of absentees in primary schools in Kita-Kyushu, Japan, in 2006.

Temporal overdispersion

It is assumed that, under the null hypothesis of no outbreaks, the number of cases N_{it} in region i ($i = 1, \ldots, m$) at some surveillance time t follows an independent negative binomial distribution $NB(\mu_{it}, \phi_{it})$ by taking the possibility of a nonnegligible time-to-time variation of Poisson mean or *temporal overdispersion* into account

$$H_0 : N_{it} \sim NB(\mu_{it}, \phi_{it})$$

where the negative binomial distribution used here is given by

$$\Pr\{N_{it} = n_{it} \mid \mu_{it}, \phi_{it}\} = \frac{\Gamma(\phi_{it} + n_{it})}{\Gamma(\phi_{it}) \, n_{it}!} \left(\frac{\phi_{it}}{\phi_{it} + \mu_{it}} \right)^{\phi_{it}} \left(\frac{\mu_{it}}{\phi_{it} + \mu_{it}} \right)^{n_{it}}$$

and

$$E(N_{it}) = \mu_{it}, \quad \mathrm{Var}(N_{it}) = \mu_{it} + \mu_{it}^2/\phi_{it} = \mu_{it} w_{it}$$

The temporal overdispersion is given by

$$w_{it} = 1 + \mu_{it}/\phi_{it}$$

and ϕ_{it} denote the parameter regulating overdispersion. Needless to say, if we do not observe any overdispersion in region i, then we have only to set $\phi_{it} = \infty$ or $w_{it} = 1$.

How to set (μ_{it}, ϕ_{it})

The expected number of cases μ_{it} and the parameter ϕ_{it} should be estimated using data from a predefined *baseline period*. If we can use the surveillance data reported for several years in the past, then we can apply an appropriate *negative binomial regression model* within the framework of generalized linear mixed models (for example, see Hardin and Hilbe, 2007; Hilbe, 2007)

$$\log E(Y_{it}) = \sum_{j=1} x_{itj}\beta_j + b_i, \quad Y_{it} \sim NB(\mu_{it}^{(Y)}, \phi_i^{(Y)})$$

where Y_{it} denotes a random variable for the observed counts data y_{it} in the predefined baseline period, x_{itj} denotes the value of covariate j such as a month, a day of the week, and so on, b_i denotes a random regional effects normally distributed with mean 0, and ϕ_{it} is usually set constant over time; i.e., $\phi_{it} = \phi_i$. This model is an extension of generalized linear mixed models by Kleinman, Lazarus, and Platt (2004) and Kleinman (2005). Using this regression model, we can set $\mu_{it} = \hat{\mu}_{it}^{(Y)}$ and $\phi_{it} = \hat{\phi}_i^{(Y)}$.

However, if the surveillance system starts quite recently, as in the case of our example illustrated later, we cannot adopt the above-stated regression approach. In this case, we can use the so-called *moving average* method. That is, it is assumed that the null expected number of cases μ_{it} is constant for each region during the *baseline period* defined, such as $\{t-1, t-2, \ldots t-B\}$ with baseline length B. Then these two parameters can be simply estimated using baseline mean $\bar{y}_{i\cdot}$ and baseline variance s_i^2 by the moment method,

$$\mu_{it} = \hat{\mu}_{it}^{(Y)} = \bar{y}_{i\cdot}$$

$$\phi_{it} = \hat{\phi}_i^{(Y)} = \begin{cases} \frac{\bar{y}_{i\cdot}^2}{s_i^2 - \bar{y}_{i\cdot}}, & \text{if } s_i^2 > \bar{y}_i \\ \infty, & \text{otherwise} \end{cases}$$

Then the alternative hypothesis is

$$H_1 : N_{it} \sim NB(\theta_{it}\mu_{it}, \phi_i), \ E(N_{it}) = \theta_{it}\mu_{it}$$

where (μ_{it}, ϕ_i) are known and θ_{it} denotes the relative risk in region i at time t.

An outbreak model

The *outbreak model*

$$\theta_{it} = \begin{cases} h(\tau + \beta_W (t - t_p + u)), & \text{if } (i,t) \in W = Z \times I_u \\ 1, & \text{otherwise} \end{cases}$$

is proposed to capture localized emerging outbreaks, where the *initial slope* of emerging outbreak that starts just after the time point $t_p - u$ within the domain W is proportional to β_W since

$$\left[\frac{\partial \theta_{it}}{\partial t} \right]_{t=t_p-u} = \beta_W h'(\tau)$$

and $h(.)$ denotes any monotonically increasing function with $h(\tau) = 1$, and the first and second differentials $h'(.)$ and $h''(.)$ are assumed to be finite. Then, the above-stated hypothesis test is simply reduced to the following hypothesis test over all possible sets of domains $W = Z \times I_u$:

$$H_0 : \beta_W = 0$$
$$H_1 : \beta_W > 0$$

Test statistics

Under the *outbreak model*, the likelihood is

$$L(\beta \mid \mu_{it}, \phi_i, t_p, u, t) = \prod_{(i,t)\in W} \frac{\Gamma(\phi_i + n_{it})}{\Gamma(\phi_i)\, n_{it}!} \left(\frac{\phi_i}{\phi_i + \theta_{it}\mu_{it}} \right)^{\phi_i} \left(\frac{\theta_{it}\mu_{it}}{\phi_i + \theta_{it}\mu_{it}} \right)^{n_{it}}$$

$$\cdot \prod_{(i,t)\in W^c} \frac{\Gamma(\phi_i + n_{it})}{\Gamma(\phi_i)\, n_{it}!} \left(\frac{\phi_i}{\phi_i + \mu_{it}} \right)^{\phi_i} \left(\frac{\mu_{it}}{\phi_i + \mu_{it}} \right)^{n_{it}}$$

Then, as with Kulldorff's space-time scan statistics, we can construct a likelihood ratio test for testing the null hypothesis $H_0 : \beta_W = 0$ against $H_1 : \beta_W > 0$. However, the likelihood ratio test statistic requires the functional form $h()$ and the maximum likelihood estimator for β_W. Therefore, we shall derive here an efficient score test that does not depend on the functional form $h()$ and does not require the maximum likelihood estimator for β_W, which is asymptotically equivalent to the likelihood ratio test. The efficient score test statistic for the null hypothesis $H_0 : \beta_W = 0$ is

$$S = \sup_{Z \in \mathscr{Z},\, 1 \leq u \leq T} \frac{\sum_{i\in Z} \sum_{t\in I_u} (n_{it} - \mu_{it})(t - t_p + u)/w_{it}}{\sqrt{\sum_{i\in Z} \sum_{t\in I_u} \mu_{it}(t - t_p + u)^2/w_{it}}}$$

Needless to say, if a Poisson distribution can be used instead of a negative binomial distribution for all regions, then we have only to set $w_{it} = 1$ for all regions. The domain $W^* = Z^* \times I_{u^*}$ for which the efficient score is maximized identifies the *most likely outbreak* (MLO), which is different from the most likely cluster. Spatial window Z can be Kulldorff's (1997) circular window or Tango and Takahashi's (2005) flexible window, or any other spatial window. In a mannner similar to Kulldorff's and Takahashi *et al.*'s space-time scan statistics, *p*-values of the most likely outbreak and secondary outbreaks are obtained through Monte Carlo hypothesis testing.

If we assume a *hot-spot cluster model* instead of the proposed *outbreak model*

$$
\theta_{it} = \begin{cases} \tau_W (> 1), & \text{if } (i,t) \in W = Z \times I_u \\ 1, & \text{otherwise} \end{cases}
$$

then the efficient score test statistic for the null hypothesis $H_0 : \tau_W = 1$ is

$$
S = \sup_{Z \in \mathcal{Z},\, 1 \leq u \leq T} \frac{\sum_{i \in Z} \sum_{t \in I_u} (n_{it} - \mu_{it}) / w_{it}}{\sqrt{\sum_{i \in Z} \sum_{t \in I_u} \mu_{it} / w_{it}}}
$$

Furthermore, a Poisson distribution can be used instead of a negative binomial distribution, and then the efficient score statistic is reduced to

$$
\begin{aligned}
S &= \sup_{Z \in \mathcal{Z},\, 1 \leq u \leq T} \frac{\sum_{i \in Z} \sum_{t \in I_u} (n_{it} - \mu_{it})}{\sqrt{\sum_{i \in Z} \sum_{t \in I_u} \mu_{it}}} \\
&= \sup_{W \in \mathcal{W}} \frac{n(W) - \mu(W)}{\sqrt{\mu(W)}}
\end{aligned}
$$

which is asymptotically equivalent to the *unconditional* likelihood ratio test in the sense that the expected number of cases $\mu(W)$ in the domain W is estimated from the baseline data.

Application

Tango and Takahashi (2008) illustrated their approaches, one with a cylindrical domain and the other with a prismatic domain, with data from a weekly surveillance of the absentees in 131 primary school districts in Kita Kyushu shi (city) during April 12 (1st week) to December 20 (30th week) in 2006 in Japan, where the total number of schoolchildren was 52,177. Figure 9.2 shows the weekly number of infectious enteritis patients in Kita Kyushu shi from April 2006 to March 2007, taken from *Infectious Disease Weekly Report* in this city, which clearly shows the occurrence of an overall outbreak during November 15 to December 20. Needless to say, there are several other reasons for students' absence from school. However, we assumed here that the proportion of absentees unrelated to infectious enteritis would be approximately constant for each primary school since the detailed data on the reason for absence were not available.

In this application, they used an eight-week moving average method to estimate the baseline information (μ_{it}, ϕ_{it}) for the analysis week t. Figure 9.3 shows the weekly number of absentees in four selected school districts, eight-week moving average line (from the 10th week, June 21), and two kinds of 95% UCLs (upper control limits) lines based on a Poisson distribution (dotted line) and the negative

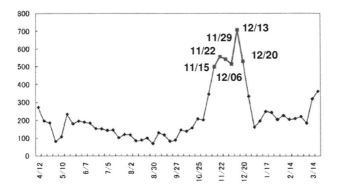

Fig. 9.2 Weekly number of infectious enteritis patients in Kita Kyushu shi from April 2006 to March 2007 in Japan (from *Infectious Disease Weekly Report* in Kita Kyushu shi).

binomial distribution (dashed-dotted line). We can observe that three school districts No. 60, No. 61, and No. 62 have nonnegligible temporal overdispersion, but school No. 63 has relatively small temporal overdispersion. We started the weekly analysis from October 11 (20th week) and continued the analysis untill December 20 (30th week), where the maximum spatial length was set as $K = 15$, the maximum temporal length was set as $T = 2$, the significance level was set as $\alpha = 0.02$, corresponding to one expected false alarm every 50 weeks or approximately 1 year (the recurrence interval, RI), and the p-value was based on the Monte Carlo hypothesis testing with $M = 999$ replicates. As *detected areas*, we considered all significant clusters (outbreaks), including significant secondary clusters (outbreaks) that do not overlap with MLC (MLO).

In what follows, we shall consider four space-time scan statistics for comparison: Kulldorff's scan statistic, Takahashi *et al.*'s scan statistic, a new scan statistic with a cylindrical domain, and a new scan statistic with a prismatic domain. We will sometimes refer to these statistics as KC, TP, PC, and PP, respectively. As it is well-known that a cylindrical scan statistic performs better than a prismatic scan statistic in detecting a circular area and the latter performs better than the former in detecting a noncircular area, our primary interest is a comparison between KC and PC and also a comparison between TP and PP.

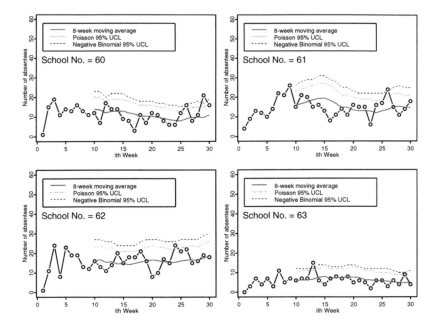

Fig. 9.3 Weekly number of absentees in four selected school districts with eight-week moving average (line) and two kinds of 95% UCLs (upper control limits) based on a Poisson distribution (dotted line) and negative binomial distribution (dashed-dotted line). Calculation of the eight-week moving average was started from the 10th week (June 21).

First, consider the comparison of the performance of two kinds of *prismatic* scan statistics. Table 9.3 summarizes the results of two prismatic scan statistics, in which we show the baseline expected number of absentees $\mu_{+t} = \sum_{i \in Z^*} \mu_{it}$ and the observed number of absentees $n_{+,t} = \sum_{i \in Z^*} n_{it}$ within the detected areas Z^* at week t. Using these statistics, we shall indicate the overall temporal trend in the number of absentees in detected areas such as

$$\left(\mu_{+,t_p} : n_{+,t_p-1} \rightarrow n_{+,t_p}\right)$$

Figure 9.4 highlights the detected areas by analysis week. For each of the analyses during October 11 to November 8, two prismatic scan statistics did not detect any areas. On November 15, when the infectious enteritis outbreak seemed to start (see Figure 9.2), PP detected three outbreaks, O_1, O_2, O_3, but TP did not, indicating an example of timely detection of outbreaks for the proposed scan statistic. For example, the detected outbreak O_1 that covered eight schools has a temporal trend ($65 : 99 \rightarrow 111$) with $p = 0.012$ and temporal length $u^* = 2$ (from November 8 to 15).

On November 22, both prismatic scan statistics detected almost the same areas, C_1 with 12 schools and O_1 with 13 schools, respectively. On November 29, only

Table 9.3 Significant clusters detected by Takahashi et al.'s *prismatic* scan statistic and significant outbreaks detected by a new *prismatic* scan statistic applied to data from weekly surveillance of the absentees in 131 primary school districts in Kita Kyushu shi, during October 11 to December 20, 2006 in Japan, where the maximum temporal length is set as $T = 2$. Bold numbers indicate the temporal period detected.

Current Week t_p	Takahashi et al.'s *prismatic* scan					A new *prismatic* scan				
	Detected areas (p-value)	No. schools Z^*	$\mu^{a)}_{+,t_p}$	$n^{a)}_{+,t_p-1}$	n_{+,t_p}	Detected areas (p-value)	No. schools Z^*	μ_{+,t_p}	n_{+,t_p-1}	n_{+,t_p}
10/11										
10/18										
10/25										
11/01										
11/08										
11/15						O_1 (0.012)	8	65	**99**	**111**
						O_2 (0.016)	11	68	**81**	**115**
						O_2 (0.018)	9	78	**114**	**117**
11/22	C_1 (0.001)	12	75	**120**	**144**	O_1 (0.003)	13	81	**123**	**155**
11/29	C_1 (0.001)	11	76	**141**	98					
12/06	C_1 (0.001)	5	33	**42**	**80**	O_1 (0.002)	7	49	**70**	**106**
12/13	C_1 (0.001)	13	93	**166**	**183**	O_1 (0.002)	12	90	**162**	**178**
						O_2 (0.003)	12	88	**121**	**159**
						O_3 (0.003)	10	53	**89**	105
						O_4 (0.003)	9	78	**90**	148
						O_5 (0.012)	11	90	**123**	142
12/20	C_1 (0.015)	2	18	**44**	36	O_1 (0.002)	10	118	**166**	193
						O_2 (0.013)	11	57	**97**	**90**

$^{a)}$ $\mu_{+,t} = \sum_{i \in Z^*} \mu_{it}$ and $n_{+,t} = \sum_{i \in Z^*} n_{it}$.

the TP statistic detected the significant area C_1 ($p = 0.001$), quite similar to the area C_1 on November 22. However, as the temporal trend ($76 : 141 \rightarrow 98$) was decreasing from the previous week, we will not consider this cluster as an outbreak. PP, on the other hand, did not detect any areas in the same week, which seems to correspond to the decreasing trend observed in the number of infectious enteritis patients. On December 6, both PP and TP detected similar areas, C_1 ($p = 0.002$) and O_1 ($p = 0.005$), respectively.

On December 13, the difference in performance of these two scan statistics was also conspicuous. This week attained the peak of the number of infectious enteritis patients. While TP detected one significant cluster C_1 ($p = 0.001$) with 13 schools with a trend ($93 : 166 \rightarrow 183$), PP detected five significant outbreaks, including the area O_1 ($p = 0.002$), which is almost the same area as C_1. All of those detected areas had an increasing trend in the number of absentees. On December 20, TP detected only one small area C_1 ($p = 0.015$) with two schools, which is a part of the area C_1 detected in the previous week, while PP detected two new areas that were not detected before, indicating a possibility of spreading to this area.

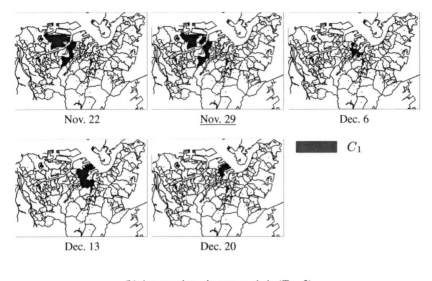

(b) A new prismatic scan statistic ($T = 2$)

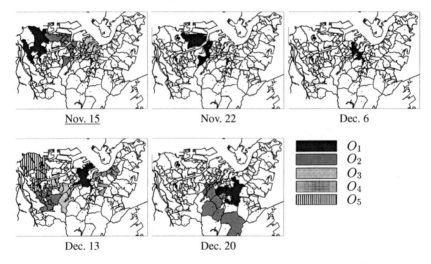

Fig. 9.4 (a) Significant clusters detected by Takahashi *et al.*'s *prismatic* scan statistic and (b) significant outbreaks detected by a new *prismatic* scan statistic applied to data from weekly surveillance of the absentees in 131 primary school districts in Kita Kyushu shi, Japan, during October 2006 to December 2006, where the maximum temporal length is set as $T = 2$.

Table 9.4 Significant clusters detected by Kuldorff's *cylindrical* scan statistic and significant outbreaks detected by a new *cylindrical* scan statistic applied to data from weekly surveillance of the absentees in 131 primary school districts in Kita Kyushu shi during October 11 to December 20, 2006 in Japan, where the maximum temporal length is set as $T = 2$. Bold numbers indicate the temporal period detected.

Current Week t_p	Takahashi *et al.*'s *prismatic* scan					A new *prismatic* scan				
	Detected areas (*p*-value)	No. schools Z^*	Baseline $\mu^{a)}_{+,t_p}$	$n^{a)}_{+,t_p-1}$	n_{+,t_p}	Detected areas (*p*-value)	No. schools Z^*	μ_{+,t_p}	n_{+,t_p-1}	n_{+,t_p}
10/11										
10/18										
10/25										
11/01										
11/08										
11/15						O_1 (0.013)	9	50	**61**	**87**
11/22	C_1 (0.001)	11	64	**101**	**130**	O_1 (0.003)	11	64	**101**	**130**
11/29	C_1 (0.001)	15	97	**168**	**116**					
12/06	C_1 (0.001)	5	32	**42**	**74**	O_1 (0.002)	5	32	**42**	**74**
	C_2 (0.004)	4	19	**30**	**44**	O_2 (0.008)	4	17	**30**	**44**
12/13	C_1 (0.001)	10	69	**130**	**141**	O_1 (0.002)	14	100	**171**	**191**
						O_2 (0.003)	14	99	**131**	**163**
						O_3 (0.008)	14	127	**159**	**200**
						O_4 (0.009)	9	75	**87**	**131**
						O_5 (0.013)	6	38	**56**	**75**
12/20	C_1 (0.001)	2	18	**44**	**36**	O_1 (0.004)	15	183	**243**	**261**
						O_2 (0.013)	14	108	**191**	**135**

$a)$ $\mu_{+,t} = \sum_{i\in Z^*} \mu_{it}$ and $n_{+,t} = \sum_{i\in Z^*} n_{it}$.

Table 9.4 show the results of two *cylindrical* scan statistics. The difference in performance of two *cylindrical* scan statistics was more or less similar to that of two *prismatic* scan statistics.

Notes

The results show that Kulldorff's and Takahashi *et al.*'s space-time scan statistics had lower power in detecting localized gradual increases in absentees compared with a new space-time scan statistic. However, we do not know the truth about what outbreaks may be present in the data we analyze, and we cannot say whether a new space-time scan statistic had a better peformance than the existing procedures. Therefore, we need an extensive simulation study to evaluate the performance of the proposed space-time scan statistic in comparison with the existing scan statistics by considering several localized emerging outbreak scenarios.

Appendix A
List of R functions

The following *R functions* are newly made for the readers of the book and are used in the Sections *Illustration with Real Data*. These functions will be made available at

http://www.niph.go.jp/soshiki/gijutsu/download/Rfunctions/index.html

- **Bithell.test**: Bithell's linear rank score test for decline trend
- **DiggleChetwynd.test**: Diggle and Chetwynd's test for spatial clustering: case-control point data
- **DiggleETAL.test**: Diggle *et al.*'s test for space-time interaction
- **Jacquez.test**: Jacquez's *k* nearest neighbors test for space-time interaction
- **KnoxA.test**: Knox's test for space-time interaction with approximated *p*-values
- **KnoxM.test**: Knox's test for space-time interaction with Monte Carlo simulated *p*-values
- **Mantel.test**: Mantel's test for space-time interaction
- **Nagarwalla.test**: Nagarwalla's scan statistic for temporal clustering
- **Stone.test**: Stone's test for decline trend
- **TangoT.index**: Tango's index for temporal clustering
- **TangoS.index**: Tango's index for spatial clustering: regional count data
- **TangoCNN.index**: Tango's index for spatial clustering: case-control point data (*k* nearest neighbors model)
- **TangoCDE.index**: Tango's index for spatial clustering: case-control point data (double exponential model)
- **TangoF.test**: Tango's score test for decline trend
- **TangoFPD.test**: Tango's score test for peak-decline trend
- **WallerLawson.test**: Waller and Lawson's score test for decline trend

References

1. Abrial D., Calavas D., Lauvergne N., Morignat E., and Ducrot C. (2003). Descriptive spatial analysis of BSE in western France. *Veterinary Research*, **34**, 749–60.
2. Alderson M.R. and Nayak R. (1971). A study of space-time clustering in Hodgkin's disease in the Manchester region. *British Journal of Preventive and Social Medicine*, **25**, 168–173.
3. Alexander F.E. (1992). Space-time clustering of childhood acute lymphoblastic leukaemia: Indirect evidence for a transmissbile agent. *British Journal of Cancer*, **65**, 589–592.
4. Alexander F.E., McKinney P.A., Moncrieff K.C., and Cartwright R.A. (1992). Residential proximity of children with leukemia and non-Hodgkins lymphoma in 3 areas of northern England. *British Journal of Cancer*, **65**, 583–588.
5. Alperovitch A., Hesse C., Lazar P., Hayat M. and Flamand R. (1974). Temporal-spatial distribution of leukaemia and haematosarcoma in seven French regions. *International Journal of Epidemiology*, **3**, 209–218.
6. Alt K.W. and Vach W. (1991). The reconstruction of "genetic kinship" in prehistoric burial complexes: Problems and statistics. In Bock H.H. and Ihm P. (Eds.), *Classification, Data Analysis, and Knowledge Organization: Models and Methods with Applications*, 299–310, Berlin: Springer-Verlag.
7. Altman D.G. (1991). *Practical Statistics for Medical Research*, London, Chapman and Hall/CRC.
8. Andrade A.L., Silva S.A., Martelli C.M., Oliveira R.M., Morais Neto O.L., Siqueira Junior J.B., Melo L.K., and Di Fabio J.L. (2004). Population-based surveillance of pediatric pneumonia: use of spatial analysis in an urban area of Central Brazil. *Cadernos de Saude Publica*, **20**, 411–421.
9. Assunção R. and Reis E.A. (1999). A new proposal to adjust Moran's *I* for population density. *Statistics in Medicine*, **18**, 2147–2162.
10. Assunção R, Costa M., Tavares A., and Ferreira S. (2006). Fast detection of arbitrarily shaped disease clusters, *Statistics in Medicine*, **25**, 723–742.
11. Bailar III J.C., Eisenberg H., and Mantel N. (1970). Time between pairs of leukemia cases, *Cancer*, **25**, 1301–1303.
12. Baker R.D. (1996). Testing for space-time clusters of unknown size. *Journal of Applied Statistics*, **23**, 543–554.
13. Bakker M.I., Hatta M., Kwenang A., Faber W.R., van Beers S.M., Klatser P.R., and Oskam L. (2004). Population survey to determine risk factors for Mycobacterium leprae transmission and infection. *International Journal of Epidemiology*, **33**, 1329–1336.
14. Barlow R.E., Bartholemew D.J., Bremner J.M. and Brunk, H.D. (1972) *Statistical Inference under Order Restrictions: the Theory and Applications of Isotonic Regression*. New York: Wiley.
15. Barton D.E., David F.N., and Herrington M. (1965). A criterion for testing contagion in time and space. *Annals of Human Genetics*, **29**, 97–103.
16. Barton D.E. and David F.N. (1966). The random intersection of two graphs. In: David F.N. (Eds.), *Research Papers in Statistics*, 45–59. New York: Wiley.
17. Berke O., Grosse Beilage E. (2003). Spatial relative risk mapping of pseudorabies-seropositive pig herds in an animal-dense region. *Journal of Veterinary Medicine*, **B50**, 322–325.
18. Besag J.E. and Newell J. (1991). The detection of clusters in rare diseases. *Journal of the Royal Statistical Society, Series A*, **154**, 143–155.
19. Besag J.E., York J.C., and Mollie A. (1991). Bayesian image restoration with two applications in spatial statistics (with discussion). *Annals of the Institute of Statistical Mathematics*, **43**, 671–681.
20. Bithell J.F. (1992). Statistical methods for analyzing point source exposures. In Elliott P., Cuzick J., English D. and Stern R. (Eds.), *Geographical and Environmental Epidemiology: Methods for Small Area Studies*, 221–230. Oxford, Oxford University Press.

21. Bithell J.F. (1995). The choice of test for detecting raised disease risk near a point source. *Statistics in Medicine*, **14**, 2309–2322.
22. Bithell J.F., Dutton S.J., Draper G.J. and Neary N.M. (1994). Distribution of childhood leukaemias and non-Hodgkin's lymphomas near nuclear installations in England and Wales. *British Medical Journal*, **309**, 501–505.
23. Bithell J.F. and Stone, R.A. (1989). On statistical methods for analysing the geographical distribution of cancer cases near nuclear installations. *J. Epidemiol. Community Health*, **43**, 79–85.
24. Bivand R. and Gebhardt A. (2000). Implementing functions for spatial statistical analysis using the R language. *Journal of Geographical Systems*, **2**, 307–317.
25. Bonetti M. and Pagano M. (2005). The interpoint distance distribution as a descriptor of point patterns, with an application to spatial disease clustering. *Statistics in Medicine*, **24**, 753–773.
26. Boyle E., Johnson H., Kelly A., and McDonnell R. (2004). Congenital anomalies and proximity to landfill sites. *Irish Medical Journal*, **97**, 16–18.
27. Breslow N. and Day N. (1987). *The Design and Analysis of Cohort Studies*, Volume 2, IARC Scientific Publication No. 82. Lyon, International Agency for Research on Cancer.
28. Broman A.T., Shun K., Munoz B., Duncan D.D. and West S.K. (2006). Spatial clustering of ocular chlamydial infection over time following treatment among households in a village in Tanzania. *Investigative Ophthalmology and Visual Science*, **47**, 99–104.
29. Carpenter T.E., Chriel M., Andersen M.M., Wulfson L., Jensen A.M., Houe H. and Greiner M. (2006). An epidemiologic study of late-term abortions in dairy cattle in Denmark, July 2000-August 2003. *Preventive Veterinary Medicine*, **77**, 215–229.
30. Centers for Disease Control and Prevention (1990a). Guidelines for investigating clusters of health events. *Morbidity and Mortality Weekly Report*, **39(RR-11)**, 1–16.
31. Centers for Disease Control and Prevention (1990b). Guidelines for investigating clusters of health events - Appendix. Summary of Methods for statistically assessing clusters of health events. *Morbidity and Mortality Weekly Report*, **39(RR-11)**, 17–23.
32. Chen R., Mantel N. and Klingberg M.A. (1984). A study of three techniques for time-space clustering in Hodgkin's disease. *Statistics in Medicine*, **3**, 173–184.
33. Childs J.E., McLafferty S.L., Sadek R., Miller G.L., Khan A.S., DuPree E.R., Advani R., Mills J.N. and Glass G. (1998). Epidemiology of roden bites and prediction of rat investigation in New York City. *American Journal of Epidemiology*, **148**, 78–87.
34. Cousens S., Smith P.G, Ward H., Everington D., Knight R.S.G, Zeidler M., Stewart G., Smith-Bathgate E.A.B, Macleod M.A, Mackenzie J., and Will R.G. (2001). Geographical distribution of variant Creutzfeldt-Jakob disease in Great Britain, 1994–2000. *Lancet*, **357**, 1002–1007.
35. Cuzick J.C. and Edwards R. (1990). Spatial clustering for inhomogeneous populations. *Journal of the Royal Statistical Society, Series B*, **52**, 73–104.
36. David F.N. and Barton D.E. (1966). Two space-time interaction tests for epidemicity. *British Journal of Social and Preventive Medicine*, **20**, 44–48.
37. Diggle P.J. (1990). A point process modelling approach to raised incidence of a rare phenomenon in the vicinity of a prespecified point. *Journal of the Royal Statistical Society, Series A*, **153**, 349–362.
38. Diggle P.J. (2003). *Statistical Analysis of Spatial Point Patterns*. London, Arnold Publishers.
39. Diggle P. and Chetwynd A. (1991). Second order analysis of spatial clustering for inhomogeneous populations. *Biometrics*, **47**, 1155–1163.
40. Diggle P.J., Chetwynd A.G., Haggkvist R. and Morris S.E. (1995). Second-order analysis of space-time clustering. *Statistical Methods in Medical Research*, **4**, 124–136.
41. Diggle P.J., Morris S., and Morton-Jones T. (1999). Case-control isotonic regression for investigation of elevation in risk around a point source. *Statistics in Medicine*, **18**, 1605–1613.
42. Diggle P.J. and Rowlingson B. (1994). A conditional approach to point process modelling of elevated risk. *Journal of the Royal Statistical Society, Series A*, **157**, 433–440.
43. Dockerty J.O., Sharples K.S., Borman B. (1999). An assessment of spatial clustering of leukemia and lymphomas among young people in New Zealand. *Journal of Epidemiology and Community Health*, **53**, 154–158.

238 A List of R functions

44. Doherr M.G., Zurbriggen A., Hett A.R., Rufenacht J. and Heim D. (2002). Geographical clustering of cases of bovine spongiform encephalopatuy (BSE) born in Switzerland after the feed ban. *The Veterinary Record*, **151**, 467–472.
45. Doi Y., Yokoyama T., Sakai M., Nakamura Y., Tango T., and Takahashi K. (2008). Spatial clusters of Creutzfeldt-Jakob disease mortality in Japan between 1995 and 2004. *Neuroepidemiology*, **30**, 222–228.
46. Dolk H., Shaddick G., Walls P., Grundy C., and Thakrar B. (1997a). Cancer incidence near radio and television transmitters in Great Britain. I. Sutton Coldfield transmitter. *American Journal of Epidemiology*, **145**, 1–9.
47. Dolk H., Elliott P., Shaddick G., Walls P., and Thakrar B. (1997b). Cancer incidence near radio and television transmitters in Great Britain. II. All high power transmitters. *American Journal of Epidemiology*, **145**, 10–17.
48. Doll R. (1978). An epidemiological perspective of the biology of cancer. *Cancer Research*, **38**, 3573–3583.
49. Donnan P.T., Parratt J.D.E., Wilson S.V., Forbes R.B., O'Riordan J.I., and Swingler R.J. (2005). Multiple sclerosis in Tayside, Scotland: detection of clusters using a spatial scan statistic. *Multiple Sclerosis*, **11**, 403–408.
50. Duczmal L. and Assunção R. (2004). A simulated annealing strategy for the detection of arbitrarily shaped clusters, *Computational Statistics and Data Analysis*, **45**, 269–286.
51. Dwass M. (1957). Modified randomization test for nonparametric hypotheses. *Annals of Mathematical Statistics*, **28**, 181–187.
52. Ederer F., Myers M.H., and Mantel N. (1964). A statistical problem in space and time: Do leukemia cases come in clusters ? *Biometrika*, **20**, 626–638.
53. Elliott P., Hills M., Beresford J., Kleinschmidt I., Jolley D., Pattenden S. et al. (1992). Incidence of cancers of the larynx and lung near incinerators of waste solvents and oils in Great Britain. *Lancet*, **339**, 854–858.
54. Elliott P., Martuzzi M., and Shaddick G. (1995). Spatial statistical methods in environmental epidemiology: A critique. *Statistical Methods in Medical Research*, **4**, 137–159.
55. Elliott P., Shaddick G., Kleinschmidt I., Jelly D., Walls P., Beresford J. and Grundy C. (1996) Cancer incidence near municipal solid waste incinerators in Great Britain. *British Journal of Cancer*, **73**, 702–710.
56. Fang Z., Kulldorff M., and Gregorio D.I.(2004). Brain cancer in the United States, 1986–95: A geographic analysis. *Neuro-Oncology*, **6**, 179–187.
57. Fang L., Yan L., Liang S., de Vlas S.J., Feng D., Han X., Zhao W., Xu B., Bian L., Yang H., Gong P., Richardus J.H., and Cao W. (2006). Spatial analysis of hemorrhagic fever with renal syndrome in China. *BMC Infectious Diseases*, **6**, 77.
58. Feller W. (1957). *An Introduction to Probability Theory and its Application*, Vol. I. Second Edition. New York: Wiley.
59. Geary R.C. (1954). The contiguity ratio and statistical mapping, *The Incorporated Statisticians*, **5**, 115–145.
60. Gilks W.R., Richardson S., and Spiegelhalter D.J. (Eds.) (1996). *Markov Chain Monte Carlo in Practice*. London: Chapman & Hall.
61. Gilman E.A. and Knox E.G. (1991). Temporal-spatial distribution of childhood leukaemia and non-Hodgkin lymphomas in Great Britain. In Draper G.J. (Eds.), *The Geographical Epidemiology of Childhood Leukaemia and Non-Hodgkin Lymphomas in Great Britain, 1966–1983*, 77–81. London: HMSO.
62. Glass A.G. and Mantel N. (1969). Lack of space-time clustering of childhood leukemia, Los Angeles county, 1960-64. *Cancer Research*, **29**, 1995–2001.
63. Glass A.G., Mantel N., Guns F.W., and Spears G.F.S. (1971). Time-space clustering of childhood leukemia in New Zealand. *Journal of the National Cancer Institute*, **47**, 329–336.
64. Glaz J., Naus J. and Wallenstein S. (2001). *Scan Statistics*. New York: Springer-Verlag.
65. Grimson R.C., Wang K.C. and Johnson P.W.C. (1981). Searching for hierarchical clusters of disease: spatial patterns of sudden infant death syndrome, *Social Science and Medicine*, **15D**, 287–293.

66. Gunz F.W. and Spears G.F.S. (1968). Distribution of acute leukaemia in time and space. Studies in New Zealand. *British Medical Journal*, **4**, 604–608.

67. Han D.W., Rogerson P.A., Nie J., Bonner M.R., Vena J.E., Vito D., Muti P., Trevisan M., Edge S.B., and Freudenheim J.L. (2004). Geographic clustering of residence in early life and subsequent risk of breast cancer (United States). *Cancer Causes and Control*, **15**, 921–929.

68. Hardin J.W. and Hilbe J.M. (2007). *Generalized Linear Models and Extensions*, Second edition. Texas: Stata Press.

69. Hedges L.V. and Olkin I. (1985). *Statistical Methods for Meta-Analysis*. London: Academic Press.

70. Heffernan R., Mostashari F., Das D., Karpati A., Kulldorff M., and Weiss D. (2004). Syndromic surveillance in public health practice, New York City. *Emerging Infectious Diseases*, **10**, 858–864.

71. Hilbe J.M. (2007). *Negative Binomial Regression*. Cambridge: Cambridge University Press.

72. Hills M. and Alexander F. (1989). Statistical methods used in assessing the risk of disease near a source of possible environmental pollution. A review. *Journal of the Royal Statistical Society, Series A*, **152**, 353–363.

73. Hjalmars U., Kulldorff M., Wahlqvist Y., and Lannering B. (1999). Increased incidence rates but no space-time clustering of childhood astrocytoma in Sweden, 1973–1992. *Cancer*, **85**, 2077–2090.

74. Huillard d'Aignaux J., Cousens S.N., Delasnerie-Laupretre N., Brandel J.P., Salomon D., Laplanche J.L., Hauw J.J., and Alperovitch A. (2002). Analysis of the geographical distribution of sporadic Creutzfeldt-Jakob disease in France between 1992 and 1998. *International Journal of Epidemiology*, **31**, 490–495.

75. Huntington R.J. and Naus J.I.(1975). A simpler expression for Kth nearest neighbor coincidence probabilities. *Annals of Probability*, **3**, 894–896.

76. Iyengar V.S. (2005). Space-time clusters with flexible shapes. *Morbidity and Mortality Weekly Report*, **54** (Supplement), 71–76.

77. Jacquez G.M. (1994). Cuzick and Edwards' test when exact locations are unknown. *American Journal of Epidemiology*, **140**, 58–64.

78. Jacquez G.M. (1996). A k nearest neighbor test for space-time interaction. *Statistics in Medicine*, **15**, 1935–1949.

79. Jennings J.M., Curriero F.C., Celentano D., and Ellen J.M. (2005). Geographic identification of high gonorrhea transmission areas in Baltimore, Maryland. *American Journal of Epidemiology*, **161**, 73–80.

80. Jung I., Kulldorff M., and Klassen A. (2007). A spatial scan statistic for ordinal data. *Statistics in Medicine*, **26**, 1594–1607.

81. Kaplan J.E., Schonberger L.B., Varano G., Jackman N., Bied J., and Gary G.W. (1982). An outbreak of acute nonbacterial gastroenteritis in a nursing home demonstration of person-to-person transmission by temporal clustering of cases. *American Journal of Epidemiology*, **116**, 940-948.

82. Klauber M.R. (1968). A study of clustering of childhood leukaemia by hospital of birth. *Cancer Research*, **28**, 1790–1792.

83. Klauber M.R. (1971). Two sample randomization test for space-time clustering. *Biometrics*, **27**: 129–142.

84. Klauber M.R. (1975). Space-time clustering tests for more than two samples. *Biometrics*, **31**, 719–726.

85. Klauber M.R. and Mustacci P. (1970). Space-time clustering of childhood leukaemia in San Francisco. *Cancer Research*, **30**, 1969–1973.

86. Klassen A., Curriero F., Kulldorff M., Alberg A.J., Platz E.A., and Neloms S.T. (2006). Missing stage and grade in Maryland prostate cancer surveillance data, 1992–1997. *American Journal of Preventive Medicine*, **30**, S77–87.

87. Kleinman K.P., Lazarus R., and Platt R. (2004). A generalized linear mixed models approach for detecting incident clusters of disease in small areas, with an application to biological terrorism. *American Journal of Epidemiology*, **159**, 217–224.

88. Kleinman K.P., Abrams A.M., Kulldorff M. and Platt R. (2005). A model-adjusted space-time scan statistic with an application to syndromic surveillance. *Epidemiology and Infection*, **133**, 409–419.

89. Knox E.G. (1959). Secular pattern of congenital oesophageal atresia. *British Journal of Preventive Social Medicine*, **13**, 222–226.

90. Knox E.G. (1964a). The detection of space-time interaction. *Applied Statistics*, **13**, 25–29.

91. Knox E.G. (1964b). Epidemiology of childhood leukemia in Northumberland and Durham. *British Journal of Preventive and Socical Medicine*, **18**, 17–24.

92. Knox E.G. and Lancashire R. (1982). Detection of minimal epidemics, *Statistics in Medicine*, **1**, 183–189.

93. Kryscio R.J., Myers M.H., Presiner S.T., Heise H.W. and Christine B.W. (1973). The space-time distribution of Hodgkin's disease in Connecticut, 1940–1969. *Journal of the National Caner Institute*, **50**, 1107–1110.

94. Kulldorff M. (1997). A spatial scan statistic, *Communications in Statistics: Theory and Methods*, **26**, 1481–1496.

95. Kulldorff M. (1998). Statistical methods for spatial epidemiology: tests for randomness. In *GIS and Health*, Gatrell A. and Loytonen M., (Eds.), 49–62. London: Taylor & Francis.

96. Kulldorff M. (2001). Prospective time periodic geographical disease surveillance using a scan statistic. *Journal of the Royal Statistical Society, Series A*, **164**, 61–72.

97. Kulldorff M., Athas W., Feuer E., Miller B., and Key C. (1998). Evaluating cluster alarms: A space-time scan statistic and brain cancer in Los Alamos. *American Journal of Public Health*, **88**, 1377–1380.

98. Kulldorff M., Heffernan R., Hartman J., Assunção R., and Mostashari F. (2005). A space-time permutation scan statistic for disease outbreak detection. *PLoS Medicine*, **2**(3), e59.

99. Kulldorff M., Huang L., Pickle L., and Duczmal L. (2006). An elliptic spatial scan statistic. *Statistics in Medicine*, **25**, 3929–3943.

100. Kulldorff M. and Hjalmars U. (1999). The Knox method and other tests for space-time interaction. *Biometrics*, **55**, 544–552.

101. Kulldorff M. and Information Management Services, Inc. (2009). SaTScan v8.0.1: Software for the spatial and space-time scan statistics. http://www.satscan.org/

102. Kulldorff M. and Nagarwalla N. (1995). Spatial disease clusters: detection and inference. *Statistics in Medicine*, **14**, 799–810.

103. Kulldorff M., Tango T., and Park P.J. (2003). Power comparisons for disease clustering tests. *Computational Statistics and Data Analysis*, **42**, 665–684.

104. Larsen R.J., Holmes C.L., and Heath C.W. (1973). A statistical test for measuring unimodal clustering: a description of the test and of its application to cases of acute leukemia in metropolitan Atlanta, Georgia. *Biometrics*, **29**, 301–309.

105. Lawson, A.B. (1993). On the analysis of mortality events associated with a prespecified fixed point. *Journal of the Royal Statistical Society, Series A*, **156**, 363–377.

106. Lawson A.B. (2008). *Bayesian Disease Mapping*. Boca Raton: CRC Press.

107. Lawson A.B., Browne W.J. and Vidal Rodeiro C.L. (2003). *Disease Mapping with WinBUGS and MLwiN*. Chichester: John Wiley & Sons.

108. Lawson, AB and Kleinman, K (Eds.) (2005). *Spatial & Syndromic Surveillance for Public Health*. Yew York: John Wiley & Sons.

109. Lawson A.B. and Viel J.F. (1995). Tests for directional space-time interaction in epidemiological data. *Statistics in Medicine*, **14**, 2380–2392.

110. Lawson A.B. and Waller L. (1996). A review of point pattern methods for spatial modelling of events around sources of pollution. *Environmetrics*, **7**, 471–488.

111. Lazarus R., Kleinman K., Dashevsky I., DeMaria A., and Platt R. (2001). Using automated medical records for rapid identification of illness syndromes (syndromic surveillance): the example of lower respiratory infection. *BMC Public Health*, **1**, 9.

112. Lazarus R., Kleinman K., Dashevsky I., Adams C., Kludt P., DeMaria A., and Platt R. (2002). Use of automated ambulatory-care encounter records for detection of acute illness clusters, including potential bioterrorism events. *Emerging Infectious Diseases*, **8**, 753–760.

113. Lloyd S. and Roberts C.J. (1973). A test for space clustering and its applications to congenital limb defects in Cardiff. *British Journal of Preventive and Social Medicine*, **27**, 186–191.

114. Lombardo J., Burkom H., Elbert E., Magruder S., Lewis S.H., Loschen W., Sari J., Sniegoski C., Wojcik R., and Pavlin J. (2003). A systems overview of the electronic surveillance system for the early notification of community-based epidemics (ESSENCE II). *Journal of Urban Health*, **80**(2), suppl.1, i32–i42.

115. Mainwaring D. (1966). Epidemiology of acute leukaemia in the Liverpool area. *British Journal of Preventive and Social Medicine*, **20**, 189–194.

116. Mantel N. (1967). The detection of disease clustering and a generalized regression approach. *Cancer Research*, **27**, 209–220.

117. Mantel N., Kryscio R.J., and Myers M.H. (1976). Tables and formulas for extended use of the Ederer-Myers-Mantel disease clustering procedure, *American Journal of Epidemiology*, **104**, 576–584.

118. Marshall R.J. (1991). A review of methods for the statistical analysis of spatial patterns of disease. *Journal of the Royal Statistical Society Series A*, **154**, 421–441.

119. McHardy J., Williams E.H., Geser A., De-The G., Beth E., and Giraldo G. (1984). Endemic Kaposi's sarcoma: Incidence and risk factors in the West Nile district of Uganda. *International Journal of Cancer*, **33**, 203–212.

120. Meighan S.S. and Knox E.G. (1965). Leukemia in childhood: Epidemiology in Oregon. *Cancer*, **18**, 811–814.

121. Michelozzi P., Capon A., Kirchmayer U., Forastiere F., Biggeri A., Barca A., ns Perlucci C.A. (2002). Adult and childhood luekemia near a high-power radio station in Rome, Italy. *American Journal of Epidemiology*, **155**, 1096–1103.

122. Molinari N., Bonaldi C., and Daures, J.P. (2001). Multiple temporal cluster detection. *Biometrics*, **57**, 577–583.

123. Moran P.A.P. (1950). Notes on continuous stochastic phenomena. *Biometrika*, **37**, 17–23.

124. Morton-Jones T., Diggle P., and Elliott P. (1999). Investigation of execss environmental risk around putative sources: Stone's test with covariate adjustment. *Statistics in Medicine*, **18**, 189–197.

125. Muirhead C. and DArby S. (1989). Royal Statistical Society meeting: Cancer near nuclear installation. *Journal of the Royal Statistical Society, Series A*, **152**, 305–384.

126. Nagarwalla N. (1996). A scan statistic with a variable window. *Statistics in Medicine*, **15**, 845–850.

127. Naus J.I. (1965). The distribution of the size of the maximum cluster of points on a line. *Journal of the American Statistical Association*, **60**, 532–538.

128. Naus J.I. (1966). Some probabilities, expectations, and variance for the size of the smallest intervals and largest clusters. *Journal of the American Statistical Association*, **61**, 1191–1199.

129. Naus J.I. and Wallenstein S. (2006). Temporal surveillance using scan statistics. *Statistics in Medicine*, **25**, 311–324.

130. O'Brien D.J., Kaneene J.B., Getis A., Lloyd J.W., Swanson G.M., and Leader R.W. (2000). Spatial and temporal comparison of selected cancers in dogs and humans, Michigan, USA, 1964–1994. *Preventive Veterinary Medicine*, **47**, 187–204.

131. Oden N. (1995). Adjusting Moran's *I* for population desnsity. *Statistics in Medicine*, **14**, 17–26.

132. Ohno Y., Aoki K., and Aoki N. (1979). A test of significance for geographic clusters of disease. *International Journal of Epidemiology*, **8**, 273–281.

133. Ohno Y. and Aoki K. (1981). Cancer deaths by city and county in Japan: a test of significance for geographic clustering of disease. *Social Science and Medicine*, **15D**, 251–258.

134. Olea-Popelka F.J., Flynn O., Costello E., McGrath G., Collins J.D., O' Keeffe J.O., Kelton D.F., Berke O., and Martin SW. (2005). Spatial relationship between Mycobacterium bovis strains in cattle and badgers in four areas in Ireland. *Preventive Veterinary Medicine*, **71**, 57–70.

135. Oliver M.N, Smith E, Siadaty M, Hauck F.R. and Pickle L.W. (2006). Spatial analysis of prostate cancer incidence and race in Virginia, 1990–1999. *American Journal of Preventive Medicine*, **30**, S67–76.

Am J Epidemiol. 2008 Dec 15;168(12):1389-96. Epub 2008 Oct 15.
Geographic clustering of nonmedical exemptions to school immunization requirements and associations with geographic clustering of pertussis.

136. Omer S.B., Enger K.S., Moulton L.H., Halsey N.A., Stokley S., and Salmon D.A. (2008). Geographic clustering of nonmedical exemptions to school immunization requirements and associations with geographic clustering of pertussis. *American Journal of Epidemiology*, **168**, 1389-1396.

137. Openshaw S., Craft A.W., Charlton M., and Birth J.M. (1988). Investigation of leukemia clusters by use of a geographical analysis machine. *Lancet*, **1**(8580), 272–273.

138. Ozonoff A., Webster T., Vieira V., Weinberg J., Ozonoff D., and Aschengrau A. (2005). Cluster detection methods applied to the Upper Cape Cod cancer data. *Environmental Health: A Global Access Science Source*, **4**, 19.

139. Patil, G.P. and Taillie C. (2004). Upper level set scan statistic for detecting arbitrarily shaped hotspots, *Environmental and Ecological Statistics*, **11**, 183–197.

140. Perez A.M., Ward M.P., Torres P., and Ritacco V. (2002). Use of spatial statistics and monitoring date to identify clustering of bovine tuberculosis in Argentina. *Preventive Veterinary Medicine*, **56**, 63–74.

141. Petridou E., Revinthi K., Alexander F.E., Haidas S., Kolouskas D., Kosmidis H., Piperopoulou F., Tzortzatou F., and Trichopoulos D. (1996). Space-time clustering of childhood leukaemia in Greece: evidence supporting a viral aetiology. *British Journal of Cancer*, **73**, 1278–1283.

142. Pfeiffer D., Robinson T., Stevenson M., Stevens K., Rogers D., and Clements A. (2008). *Spatial Analysis in Epidemiology*. New York: Oxford University Press.

143. Pike M.C. and Smith P.G. (1968). Disease clustering: a generalization of Knox's approach to the detection of space-time interactions. *Biometrics*, **24**, 541–546.

144. Pike M.C. and Smith P.G. (1974). A case-control approach to examine diseases for evidence of contagion, including diseases with long latent periods. *Biometrics*, **30**, 263–279.

145. Pinkel D. and Nefzger D. (1959). Some epidemiological features of childhood leukemia in the Buffalo, NY area. *Cancer*, **12**, 351–357.

146. Pinkel D., Dawd J.E., and Bross I.D.J. (1963). Some epidemiological features of malignant solid tumors of children in the Buffalo, NY area. *Cancer*, **16**, 28–33.

147. Platt R., Bocchino C., Caldwell B., Harmon R., Kleinman K., Lazarus R., Nelson, A.F., Nordin J.D., and Ritzwoller P. (2003). Syndromic surveillance using minimum transfer of identifiable data: the example of the National Bioterrorism Syndromic Surveilance Demonstration Program. *Journal of Urban Health*, **80** (2), suppl.1, i25–i31.

148. Polack S.R., Solomon A.W., Alexander N.D.E., Massae P.A., Safari S., Shao J.F., Foster A., and Mabey D.C.(2005). The household distribution of trachoma in a Tanzanian village: an application of GIS to the study of trachoma. *Transactions of the Royal Society of Tropical Medicine and Hygiene*, **99**, 218–225.

149. Pollack L.A., Gotway C.A., Bates J.H., Parikh-Patel A., Richards T.B., Seeff L.C., Hodges H., and Kassim S. (2006). Use of the spatial scan statistic to identify geographic variations in late stage colorectal cancer in California. *Cacer Causes and Control*, **17**, 449–457.

150. Pugliatti M., Riise T., Sotgiu M.A., Satta W.M., Sotgiu S., Pirastru M.I., and Rosati G. (2006). Evidence of early childhood as the susceptibility period in multiple sclerosis: Space-time cluster analysis in a sardinian population. *American Journal of Epidemiology*, **164**, 326-333.

151. Ripley B.D. (1976). The second-order analysis of stationary point processes. *Journal of Applied Probability*, **13**, 255–266.

152. Ripley B.D. (1977). Modelling spatial patterns (with discussion). *Journal of the Royal Statistical Society, Series B*, **39**, 172–212.

153. Roberts C.H., Laurence K.M., and Lloyd S. (1975). An investigation of space and space-time clustering in a large sample of infants with neural tube defects born in Cardiff. *British Journal of Preventive and Social Medicine*, **29**, 202–204.

154. Rogerson P. (1999). The detection of clusters using a spatial version of the chi-squared goodness-of-fit test. *Geographical Analysis*, **31**, 130–147.

155. Rogerson P. (2006). Statistical methods for the detection of spatial clustering in case-control data. *Statistics in Medicine*, **25**, 811–823.
156. Rowlingson B. and Diggle P. (1993). Splancs: spatial point pattern analysis code in S-Plus. *Computers and Geosciences*, **19**, 627–655.
157. Shaddick G. and Elliott P. (1996). Use of Stone's method in studies of disease risk around point sources of environmental pollution. *Statistics in Medicine*, **15**, 1927–1934.
158. Sheehan T.J. and De Chello (2005). A space-time analysis of the proportion of late stage breast cancer in Massachusetts, 1988 to 1997. *International Journal of Heath Geographics*, **4**, 15.
159. Siemiatycki J. (1978). Mantel's space-time clustering statistic: computing higher moments and a comparison of various data transforms. *Journal of Statistical Computation and Simulation*, **7**, 13–31.
160. Smith P.G. and Pike M.C. (1974). A note on a "close pairs" test for space clustering. *British Journal of Preventive and Social Medicine*, **28**, 63–64.
161. Smith P.G., Pike M.C., Till M.M., and Hardisty R.M. (1976). Epidemiology of childhood leukaemia in Greater London: a search for evidence of transmission assuming a possibly long latent period. *British Medical Journal*, **33**, 1–8.
162. Smith K.L., DeVos V., Bryden H., Price L.B., Hugh-Jones, M.E., and Keim P. (2000). Bacillus anthracis diversity in Kruger National Park. *Journal of Clinical Microbiology*, **38**, 3780–3784.
163. Snow J. (1854). *On the Mode of Communication of Cholera*. Second edition. London: Churchill Livingsone.
164. Sonesson C. and Bock D. (2003). A review and discussion of prospective statistical surveillance in public health. *Journal of the Royal Statistical Society, Series A*, **166**, 5–21.
165. Song C. and Kulldorff M. (2003). Power evaluation of disease clustering tests. *International Journal of Health Geographics*, **2**, 9.
166. Song C. and Kulldorff M. (2005). Tango's maximized excess events test with different weights. *International Journal of Health Geographics*, **4**, 32.
167. Stone, R.A. (1988). Investigation of excess environmental risks around putative sources: statistical problems and a proposed test. *Statistics in Medicine*, **7**, 649–660.
168. Takahashi K., Kulldorff M., Tango T., and Yih K. (2008). A flexibly shaped space-time scan statistic for disease outbreak detection and monitoring. *International Journal of Health Geographics* **7**, 14.
169. Takahashi K. and Tango T. (2006). An extended power of cluster detection tests. *Statistics in Medicine*, **25**, 841–852.
170. Takahashi K., Yokoyama T., and Tango T. (2009). *FleXScan: Software for the Flexble Spatial Scan Statistic*. v3.0. National Institute of Public Health, Japan.
http://www.niph.go.jp/soshiki/gijutsu/index_e.html/
171. Tango T. (1984). The detection of disease clustering in time. *Biometrics*, **40**, 15–26.
172. Tango T. (1990). Asymptotic distribution of an index for disease clustering. *Biometrics*, **46**, 351–357.
173. Tango T. (1995). A class of tests for detecting "general" and "focused" clustering of rare diseases. *Statistics in Medicine*, **14**, 2323–2334.
174. Tango, T. (1999). Comparison of general tests for disease clustering, In *Disease Mapping and Risk Assessment for Public Health*, (Lawson A.B. *et al.*, Eds.), 111–117. New York: Wiley & Sons.
175. Tango T. (2000). A test for spatial disease clustering adjusted for multiple testing. *Statistics in Medicine*, **19**, 191–204.
176. Tango T. (2002). Score tests for detecting excess risks around putative sources. *Statistics in Medicine*, **21**, 497–514.
177. Tango T. (2007). A class of multiplicity adjusted tests for spatial clustering based on case-control point data. *Biometrics*, **63**, 119–127.
178. Tango T. (2008). A spatial scan statistic with s restricted likelihood ratio, *Japanese Journal of Biometrics*, **29**, 75–95.

179. Tango T., Fujita T., Tanihata T., Minowa M., Doi Y., Kato N., Kunikane S., Uchiyama I., Tanaka M., and Uehata T. (2004). Risk of adverse reproductive outcomes associated with proximity to municipal solid waste incinerators with high dioxin emission levels in Japan. *Journal of Epidemiology*, **14**, 83–93.

180. Tango T. and Takahashi K. (2005). A flexibly shaped spatial scan statistic for detecting clusters. *International Journal of Health Geographics*, **4**, 11. http://www.ij-healthgeographics.com/content/4/1/11

181. Tango T. and Takahashi K. (2008). A new space-time scan statistic for timely outbreak detection taking overdispersion into account. The 7th Annual International Society for Disease Surveillance Conference, December 3–5, 2008, Raleigh, North Carolina.

182. Till M.M., Hardisty R.M., Pike M.C., and Doll R. (1967). Childhood leukaemia in Greater London: a search for evidence of clustering. *British Medical Journal*, **3**, 755–758.

183. Turnbull B.W., Iwano E.J., Burnnett W.S., Howe H.L., and Clark L.C. (1990). Monitoring for clusters of disease: Application to leulemia incidence in upstate New York. *American Journal of Epidemiology*, **132**, suppl. S136–143.

184. Van Steensel-Moll H.A., Valkenburg H.A., Vandenbrowke H.J.P., and Van Zanen G.E. (1983). Time space distribution of childhood leukemia in the Netherlands. *Journal of Epidemiology and Community Health*, **37**, 145–148.

185. Viel J.F., Arveux P., Baverel J., and Cahn J.Y. (2000). Soft-tissue sarcoma and non-Hodgkin's lymphoma clusters around a municpal solid waste incinerator with high dioxin emission levels. *American Journal of Epidemiology*, **152**, 13–19.

186. Viel J.F., Floret N., and Mauny F. (2005). Spatial and space-time scan statistics to detect low clusters of sex ratio. *Environmental and Ecological Statistics*, **12**, 289–299.

187. Waldhor T. (1996). The spatial autocorrelation coefficient Moran's I under heteroscedasticity. *Statistics in Medicine*, **15**, 887–892.

188. Wallenstein S. (1980). A test for detection of clustering over time, *American Journal of Epidemiology*, **111**, 367–372.

189. Wallenstein S. and Neft N. (1987). An approximation for the distribution of the scan statistic. *Statistics in Medicine*, **6**, 197–207.

190. Waller, L.A. (1996). Statistical power and design of focused clustering studies, *Statistics in Medicine*, **15**, 765–782.

191. Waller L.A. and Gotway C.A. (2004). *Applied Spatial Statistics for Public Health Data*. New York: John Wiley & Sons.

192. Waller, L.A. and Lawson, A.B. (1995). The power of focused tests to detecet disease clustering. *Statistics in Medicine*, **14**, 2291–2308.

193. Waller L.A., Turnbull B.W., Clark L.C., and Nasca P. (1992). Chronic disease surveillance and testing of clustering of disease and exposure: Application to leukemia incidence and TCE-contaminated dumpsites in upstate New York. *Environmetrics*, **3**, 281–300.

194. Waller L.A., Turnbull B.W., Clark L.C., and Nasca P. (1994). Spatial pattern analysis to detect rare clusters. In Lange N., Ryan L., Billard L., Brillinger D., Conquest L., and Greenhouse J (Eds.), *Case Studies in Biometry*, 3–23. New York: Wiley.

195. Walter S.D. (1992a). The analysis of regional patterns in health data: I. Distributional considerations. *American Journal of Epidemiology*, **136**, 730–741.

196. Walter S.D. (1992b). The analysis of regional patterns in health data: II. The power to detect environmental effects. *American Journal of Epidemiology*, **136**, 742–759.

197. Wartenberg D. and Greenberg M. (1990). Detecting disease clusters: the importance of statistical power. *American Journal of Epidemiology*, **132** supple., S156–166.

198. Weinstock M.A. (1981). A generalized scan statistic test for the detection of clusters, *International Journal of Epidemiology*, **10**, 289–293.

199. Whittemore A.S. and Keller J.B. (1986). A letter to the editor. On Tango's index of disease clustering in time. *Biometrics*, **42**, 218.

200. Whittemore A.S., Friend N., Brown B.W., and Holly E.A. (1987). A test to detect clusters of disease. *Biometrika*, **74**, 631–635.

Index

A

additive excess risk model   184
aggregated pattern   11

B

Baker's Max test   154, 162, 168
Bayes' theorem   40
Bayesian model   35, 40
   hierarchical   44
Besag and Newell's test   79, 190
birth cluster   4
Bithell's linear risk score test   187, 192, 198, 209
bivariate power distribution   103, 106, 107, 109–111

C

CAR model   46, 91
cell-occupancy distribution   56
CEPP, cluster evaluation permutation procedure   79
choropleth map   34
circular window   23
clinal cluster   22, 25
cluster   9
cluster detection tests   4
clustering   9
clustering index   54
complete spatial randomness   13
conditional autoregressive model   46
conditional tests   184, 191
conjugate prior   40
critical space limit   151
critical time limit   151

Cuzick

Cuzick and Edwards' test   27, 116, 119, 129
cylindrical hot-spot cluster   219, 225

D

death cluster   4
decline hypothesis   185
Diggle and Chetwynd's test   125, 137, 144
Diggle et al.'s test   157, 164, 177
Diggle, Morris, and Morton-Jones' test   186, 195, 205
direct standardization   35
disease mapping   33
disjoint statistic   52
DSR, directly standardized mortality rate   36

E

eccentricity penalty   85
Ederer, Myers, and Mantel's method   52
Ederer-Myers-Mantel's method   56
efficient score test   227
empirical Bayes estimate   41, 43

F

flexibly shaped window   81
FleXScan   7
focused tests   3, 181
full Bayes estimate   42

G

GAM, geographical analysis machine   78
gamma distribution   40
Geary's contiguity ratio c 75
general tests   3

GLMM, generalized linear mixed model
213, 222
global clustering tests   3

H

hot-spot cluster   22, 25
hyperparameters   42
hyperprior distributions   42

I

indirect standardization   35
ISR, indirectly standardized mortality rate
36

J

Jacquez's test   155, 163, 171, 173

K

K-function   13, 14, 118
    diagnostic plots   166
    edge correction term   14
    edge-corrected estimator   13
    space and time   157, 165
Knox's test   151, 160, 168, 170
    Barton and David's formula of variance
    160
    Kulldorff and Hjalmars's Approach   167
Kulldorff's scan statistic
    cylindrical space-time   211, 215, 216, 219,
        222, 223
        permutation   217
    focused test   190, 201
    spatial scan statistic
        case-control point data   128
        circular   80, 88, 94, 101
        elliptic version   85
    temporal clustering   55, 59, 69

L

likelihood ratio   60
likelihood ratio test   58
log-normal model   44

M

Mantel's test   152, 161, 171, 173
maximum temporal length   216
measure of closeness   23, 26, 54, 77
    clinal type   24, 153, 162

double exponential   77
double exponential clinal model   117
hot-spot model   118
hot-spot type   23, 151
MEET, maximized excess events test   78, 86
MLC, most likely cluster   80, 88, 227
MLO, most likely outbreak   227
Monte Carlo hypothesis testing   29
Moran's *I*   75
moving average   226
multinomial distribution   52
multiple testing   80

N

Nagarwalla's scan statistic   58, 63
Naus' scan statistic   57, 62
nearest neighbors   27, 28, 116, 120
negative binomial distribution   41, 225
negative binomial regression model   226
noninformative priors   44
null expected number of cases   183
    conditional   74, 184, 213, 215, 225
        covariate-adjusted   74
    unconditional   183, 225

O

onset cluster   4
Openshaw *et al.*'s geographical analysis
    machine   78
outbreak model   226

P

peak-decline hypothesis   185
Pointwise tolerance limits   127
Poisson distribution   17, 38
Poisson generalized likelihood ratio   218
Poisson-gamma model   40, 41
pool-adjacent violators algorithm   186, 191
population growth rate   159, 179
posterior distribution   40
prior distribution   40
prismatic hot-spot cluster   220

R

R   6
random labeling hypothesis   116, 196
random pattern   9
recurrence interval   218
regular pattern   10
relative risk   38

Bayes estimator   40
CAR model-based full Bayes estimate   47
empirical Bayes estimator   41, 42
fixed-effects   39
full Bayes estimator   42
log-normal model-based full Bayes estimate   46
marginal maximum likelihood estimator   41, 42
maximum likelihood estimator   39
random-effects   40
restricted likelihood ratio   85
Rogerson's standardized excess events test, SEET   78

S

SaTScan   6
scan statistic   53
secondary clusters   81
simulated p-value   30
smoothed disease maps   35
SMR, standardized mortality ratio   15, 34, 71, 91, 185
space-time clustering   2, 150
space-time interaction   150, 157
space-time scan statistic   211
spatial autocorrelation   30, 44, 46
spatial clustering   2, 33, 71
   case-control point data   113
spatial pattern   9
spatial point process   12
   first-order measure   13
   homogeneous   12
   homogeneous Poisson process   12, 13
   inhomogeneous Poisson process   14, 16
   isotropy   12
   second-order measure   13
   stationarity   12
spatial scan statistic   80
spatial-temporal Poisson process   157
Splancs   7
standard population   35

standardization   35
Stone's test   185, 191, 197, 209
syndromic surveillance   216, 222

T

Takahashi *et al.*'s prismatic space-time scan statistic   217, 220, 222, 223
Tango and Takahashi's flexible spatial scan statistic   81, 89, 97
Tango's excess events test
   EET   77
Tango's index   25
   spatial clustering
      case-control point data   121, 122, 130, 134, 141
      regional count data   55, 77, 86, 92, 101
   temporal clustering   55, 60, 65, 68
Tango's maximized excess events test, MEET   78, 86
Tango's score test
   decline trend   189, 193, 199, 209
   peak-decline trend   190, 194, 200, 209
Tango's spatial scan statistic
   restricted likelihood ratio   90, 99
temporal clustering   2, 49
temporal overdispersion   225
Turnbull *et al.*'s cluster evaluation permutation procedure   79

U

unconditional tests   184
upper level set   81

W

Wallenstein and Neff's approximation   53, 58, 63
Waller and Lawson's score test   187, 192, 199, 209
Whittemore *et al.*'s test   76

Breinigsville, PA USA
13 May 2010
237919BV00005B/17/P